HEALTH, TASTE, AVOCADO WISDOM

Health, Taste, Avocado Wisdom

Solomon Raj

Noble Publishing

Contents

1. INDEX — 1
2. Chapter 1 — 3
3. Chapter 2 — 22
4. Chapter 3 — 48
5. Chapter 4 — 71
6. Chapter 5 — 93
7. Chapter 6 — 113
8. Chapter 7 — 136

1

INDEX

Chapter 1: Introduction to Avocado Bliss

1.1 Overview of avocados as a versatile superfood

1.2 Historical significance and cultural importance

1.3 Brief exploration of health benefits

Chapter 2: The Nutrient Powerhouse

2.1 In-depth examination of the nutritional profile of avocados

2.2 How avocados contribute to overall health and well-being

2.3 Exploring the impact on weight management and cardiovascular health

Chapter 3: Culinary Delights: Avocado in Every Bite

3.1 Creative and delicious avocado recipes

3.2 Avocado's role in enhancing taste and texture in various dishes

3.3 Tips for incorporating avocados into different cuisines

Chapter 4: A Taste of Avocado Wisdom

4.1 Connecting mindfulness and nutrition

4.2 The joy of savoring each bite mindfully

4.3 Cultivating a healthy relationship with food through avocado wisdom

Chapter 5: Avocado in Traditional Medicine

5.1 Historical uses of avocados in traditional healing practices

5.2 Modern scientific perspectives on the medicinal properties of avocados

5.3 Integrating avocado wisdom into holistic well-being

Chapter 6: Growing Your Own Avocado Tree

6.1 A guide to cultivating avocados at home

6.2 Sustainable practices and environmental benefits

6.3 Connecting with nature through avocado cultivation

Chapter 7: Avocado Lifestyle: Nurturing Body and Soul

7.1 The holistic approach to health and well-being

7.2 Building a balanced lifestyle with avocados at its core

7.3 Personal stories and testimonials of individuals who have embraced the avocado lifestyle

2

Chapter 1

Introduction to Avocado Bliss

In the huge embroidered artwork of culinary joys, one humble natural product has ascended to noticeable quality, catching the hearts and palates of food devotees overall — the avocado. Its excursion from a local delicacy to a worldwide sensation is a demonstration of the developing preferences of present day culture and the culinary speculative chemistry that changes basic fixings into gastronomic miracles.

The avocado, logically known as Persea History of the U.S, is a natural product local to South Focal Mexico. Having a place with the Lauraceae family, this pear-molded green diamond has risen above its geological roots to turn into an image of solid residing and complex eating. As of late, it has procured a put on the platform of superfoods, lauded for its supplement rich structure and flexible applications in the kitchen.

The charm of avocados lies not just in their velvety surface and gentle, rich flavor yet in addition in their nourishing profile. These natural products are a rich wellspring of monounsaturated fats, which are considered heart-solid and add to the general prosperity of the shopper. Avocados likewise gloat a plenty of nutrients and minerals, including potassium, vitamin K, vitamin E, and different B-nutrients.

As the world turns out to be more wellbeing cognizant, avocados have turned into a go-to decision for those looking for supplement thick, entire food choices. The ascent of wellbeing patterns and the accentuation on careful eating have pushed the avocado into the spotlight, making it a staple fixing in a horde of dishes — from servings of mixed greens and sandwiches to smoothies and treats.

Past its wholesome benefits, the avocado has cut a specialty for itself in the culinary scene because of its striking flexibility. Its unpretentious flavor profile permits it to flawlessly coordinate into both appetizing and sweet arrangements, adjusting to different foods and culinary styles. From conventional guacamole in Mexican food to vanguard avocado frozen yogurt in trial kitchens, the potential outcomes are pretty much as boundless as the creative mind of culinary experts all over the planet.

One can't talk about the avocado peculiarity without recognizing the online entertainment upheaval's job in moving it to fame. The visual allure of the dynamic green tissue, whether cut, crushed, or cunningly organized, has made avocados a most loved subject for food bloggers and Instagram powerhouses. The hashtag #avocado has amassed large number of posts, making a virtual local area limited by a common appreciation for this striking natural product.

The avocado toast pattern, portrayed by a basic yet rich mix of cut avocado on toasted bread, has turned into a social standard. Its notoriety has risen above breakfast menus, turning into an image of a wellbeing cognizant and knowing way of life. Avocado-driven diners have grown in metropolitan places, offering a variety of avocado-implanted dishes that take care of the developing interest for new, healthy, and stylishly satisfying dinners.

The avocado's excursion from indefinite quality to universality isn't without its difficulties. The flood in worldwide interest has prompted ecological worries, especially in districts where avocado development is a significant industry. The ecological effect of water-serious avocado ranches and deforestation for horticultural development has started banters about the moral utilization of this adored organic product.

Notwithstanding these difficulties, the avocado's social importance couldn't possibly be more significant. It has turned into an image of innovation, wellbeing, and culinary development. Its presence on menus isn't just a culinary decision however an impression of developing buyer inclinations and the harmonious connection among food and culture.

To genuinely see the value in the avocado's effect, one should dive into its rich history and social importance. The avocado's excursion from a staple in the eating routine of old Mesoamerican developments to a worldwide sensation is a story of versatility, flexibility, and diverse trade.

The avocado's underlying foundations can be followed back to pre-Columbian times, where it assumed a crucial part in the eating regimens of civic establishments like the Aztecs and the Maya. Known as "ahuacatl" in the Nahuatl language, the avocado held an exceptional spot in these social orders, both as a food source and an image of fruitfulness and overflow. The Aztecs even accepted that avocados had Spanish fly characteristics, further upgrading their social importance.

Spanish wayfarers experiencing avocados during their movements in the fifteenth and sixteenth hundreds of years assumed a urgent part in acquainting the natural product with the more extensive world. The pilgrims were captivated by this extraordinary green products of the soil its true capacity as a significant food source. The avocado's excursion from the Americas to Europe denoted the start of its worldwide scattering.

The avocado tracked down a responsive crowd in nations with reasonable environments for development, like Spain and Portugal. Over the long run, it spread to different regions of the planet, including Africa, Asia, and ultimately North America. The flexibility of the avocado tree to various ecological circumstances added to its fruitful coordination into assorted rural scenes.

In the US, the avocado's notoriety started to take off in the mid twentieth 100 years. California arose as a central member in avocado development, with the state's Mediterranean-like environment demonstrating ideal for the natural product bearing trees. The Hass avocado, a cultivar with an unmistakable pebbly skin and smooth surface, turned into the perfect example for avocados in the U.S. market.

The avocado's excursion from a local delicacy to a standard fixing was not without challenges. During the twentieth 100 years, avocados confronted doubt because of their high fat substance, a healthful quality that become undesirable during the time of low-fat weight control plans. Nonetheless, as nourishing science developed, the impression of solid fats moved, and avocados recovered their status as a nutritious and healthy food decision.

The late twentieth century saw the avocado's rising to fame, powered by changing culinary patterns and a developing consciousness of the significance of entire, supplement thick food sources. Avocado-driven recipes multiplied in cookbooks and culinary magazines, catching the minds of home cooks and expert gourmet specialists the same.

The 21st century introduced another period for the avocado, set apart by its change into a social symbol. The ascent of online entertainment stages, especially Instagram, assumed a vital part in molding the avocado's picture as an attractive and shareable food. The visual allure of avocado-driven dishes turned into a main thrust behind their ubiquity, transforming the organic product into an online entertainment sensation.

The avocado toast pattern, which picked up speed in the mid 2010s, embodied the combination of straightforwardness and complexity that characterizes present day culinary style. The fundamental blend of ready avocado on toasted bread turned into a material for culinary inventiveness, with fixings going from poached eggs and cherry tomatoes to radishes and bean stew drops. Avocado toast turned into a worldwide peculiarity, rising above geological and social limits.

The avocado's social importance stretches out past its culinary applications. It has turned into an image of a wellbeing cognizant and ecologically mindful way of life. The interest for avocados, frequently named "green gold," has driven financial development in locales where development is a significant industry. Be that as it may, this monetary aid has additionally raised moral worries in regards to the ecological effect of huge scope avocado cultivating.

One of the essential difficulties related with avocado development is its water utilization. Avocado trees are water-escalated, and in districts confronting water shortage, this has brought up issues about the manageability of enormous scope avocado cultivating. Also, the extension of avocado plantations has been connected to deforestation in certain areas, prompting natural surroundings misfortune and ecological debasement.

The moral problem encompassing avocados has provoked conversations about capable utilization and the requirement for feasible agrarian practices. Customers, gourmet specialists, and policymakers the same are wrestling with the situation of partaking in a darling natural product while guaranteeing that its creation lines up with ecological and social qualities.

As the avocado keeps on molding culinary scenes and buyer inclinations, it likewise fills in as a mirror reflecting more extensive cultural patterns. The avocado's excursion from a neighborhood delicacy to a worldwide peculiarity exemplifies the unique transaction between culture, trade, and soul. Its story is one of variation, advancement, and the developing connection among humankind and the food we hold dear.

1.1 Overview of avocados as a versatile superfood

In the domain of superfoods, few have accomplished the broad approval and love presented to the avocado. This unpretentious green organic product, with its smooth, rich surface and gentle, rich flavor, has risen above its starting points to turn into a culinary peculiarity and a dietary force to be reckoned with. The avocado's excursion from a territorial specialty to a worldwide most loved is a demonstration of its flexibility, healthful lavishness, and the developing preferences of knowing purchasers.

Naturally delegated Persea History of the U.S, the avocado is local to South Focal Mexico, where it has been developed for millennia. Its development originates before the appearance of Europeans in the Americas, and the natural product held an extraordinary spot in the eating regimens and societies of old Mesoamerican civilizations. Known by different names, including "ahuacatl" in Nahuatl, the avocado was a wellspring of food as well as an image of richness and overflow.

What separates the avocado as a superfood is its supplement thick creation. While certain natural products are basically wellsprings of starches, avocados stand apart because of their high happy of monounsaturated fats — the heart-sound fats likewise tracked down in olive oil. This particular fat profile, joined with a variety of fundamental nutrients and minerals, makes avocados a dietary force to be reckoned with.

One of the champion highlights of avocados is their rich substance of monounsaturated unsaturated fats, especially oleic corrosive. These solid fats have been related with different medical advantages, including further developed heart wellbeing and a decreased gamble of cardiovascular infections. The utilization of monounsaturated fats is frequently suggested as a feature of a reasonable eating regimen, and avocados give a scrumptious and fulfilling method for integrating these fats into dinners.

Avocados are likewise a brilliant wellspring of potassium, a fundamental mineral that assumes a vital part in keeping up with legitimate heart and muscle capability. Sufficient potassium admission is related with lower pulse levels, and remembering avocados for the eating routine can add to meeting everyday potassium prerequisites.

Notwithstanding potassium, avocados supply a variety of fundamental nutrients. Vitamin K, significant for blood coagulating and bone wellbeing, is available in overflow. Avocados additionally contain vitamin E, a cancer prevention agent that shields cells from harm brought about by free revolutionaries. The B-nutrient family, including B5, B6, and folate, is very much addressed in avocados, supporting different physical processes like energy digestion and the arrangement of red platelets.

The nourishing profile of avocados makes them an important expansion to a reasonable and wellbeing cognizant eating regimen. The mix of solid fats, nutrients, and minerals gives fundamental supplements as well as adds to a sensation of satiety and fulfillment. This satisfying quality makes avocados a useful part for those hoping to oversee weight or keep a smart dieting schedule.

Past their dietary substance, avocados have acquired their superfood status through their surprising adaptability in the kitchen. Not at all like many natural products that are restricted to sweet applications, avocados flawlessly incorporate into both exquisite and sweet dishes, offering a wide material for culinary innovativeness.

One of the most notorious and broadly embraced ways of getting a charge out of avocados is as guacamole — an exemplary Mexican dish that has turned into a worldwide number one. Pounded avocados joined with fixings like lime juice, onions, tomatoes, and cilantro make a lively and tasty plunge that matches well with tortilla chips or fills in as a sauce for tacos and different dishes.

The avocado's versatility stretches out past customary recipes to embrace inventive culinary manifestations. Avocado toast, a pattern that picked up speed during the 2010s, is a perfect representation of how a basic mix can develop into a social sensation. The fundamental reason — ready avocado spread on toasted bread — fills in as an establishment for vast varieties, with fixings going from poached eggs and smoked salmon to feta cheddar and cherry tomatoes.

Avocado's smooth surface makes it an optimal possibility for consolidation into smoothies and sweets. Mixing avocados with organic products, yogurt, and other healthy fixings yields velvety and nutritious treats. Avocado chocolate mousse, for example, has turned into a famous option in contrast to customary mousse recipes, exhibiting the organic product's capacity to improve both surface and healthy benefit.

The ascent of plant-based counts calories and the mission for meat options have additionally raised avocados' status. As a plant-based wellspring of solid fats and supplements, avocados assume an essential part in gathering the dietary necessities of those deciding on veggie lover or vegetarian ways of life. Avocado cuts as often as possible track down their direction into sandwiches, mixed greens, and wraps, giving a wonderful and nutritious substitute for creature based fats.

In the realm of culinary advancement, gourmet experts and home cooks the same keep on investigating the limits of avocado's flexibility. From avocado fries and avocado-lime sorbet to avocado-injected mixed drinks, the natural product's true capacity appears to be boundless. The eagerness to explore different avenues regarding avocados mirrors a more extensive change in shopper inclinations toward new, entire food varieties that offer both flavor and nourishing advantages.

The avocado's excursion from a provincial delicacy to a worldwide superfood is unpredictably attached to the changing scene of dietary inclinations and culinary patterns. The ascent of health culture, with its accentuation on careful eating and supplement thick food varieties, has impelled avocados into the spotlight. The natural product's capacity to line up with assorted dietary examples, including ketogenic, paleo, and Mediterranean weight control plans, has additionally added to its general allure.

Online entertainment plays had a vital impact in enhancing the avocado's range and impact. Instagram, specifically, has turned into a stage where the visual allure of avocados becomes the dominant focal point.

The lively green tints of cut avocados, the sly plan of avocado dishes, and the inventive blends exhibited by food bloggers and powerhouses have transformed the hashtag #avocado into a virtual festival of this darling organic product.

The avocado toast pattern, frequently embellished with tastefully satisfying fixings, has turned into a social standard. Past its culinary benefits, the dish has turned into an image of a specific way of life — a way of life that values wellbeing, taste, and a hint of complexity. Avocado-driven restaurants, profiting by this pattern, have grown in metropolitan places, offering menus that exhibit the organic product's flexibility in different culinary styles.

While the avocado's ubiquity keeps on taking off, its process isn't without challenges. The flood in worldwide interest for avocados has raised ecological and moral worries, especially in districts where development is a significant industry. The water-serious nature of avocado cultivating, combined with issues of deforestation and living space misfortune, has incited a reexamination of the maintainability of avocado creation.

Buyers, cooks, and policymakers are progressively aware of the ecological impression related with the avocados they appreciate. Conversations about dependable obtaining, feasible cultivating practices, and fair work conditions are becoming fundamental to the avocado story. Adjusting the craving for a darling and nutritious natural product with the need to limit environmental effect stays a perplexing and continuous test.

All in all, the avocado's development from a neighborhood delicacy to a worldwide superfood mirrors the complex exchange between nourishment, culinary imagination, and social patterns. Its ascent to popularity isn't only a consequence of its scrumptious taste and dietary lavishness yet in addition a demonstration of its flexibility and adaptability in the kitchen. As buyers keep on looking for healthy, tasty, and outwardly engaging food varieties, the avocado stands ready to keep up with its status as a darling and getting through image of sound living and gastronomic development.

1.2 Historical significance and cultural importance

The avocado, with its velvety tissue and particular flavor, is something beyond a culinary pleasure; it conveys with it a rich embroidery of verifiable importance and social significance. To genuinely see the value in the avocado's excursion, one should dig into its foundations in old Mesoamerican developments, where it was a dietary staple as well as an image of social and otherworldly importance.

The account of the avocado starts in the district that is presently South Focal Mexico, where the natural product's development can be followed back millennia. The Aztecs, perhaps of the most unmistakable

Mesoamerican development, assumed an essential part in the early development and enthusiasm for avocados.

They alluded to the organic product as "ahuacatl," a word that connoted the natural product as well as bore an optional importance — gonad, a sign of approval for the avocado's shape. This double significance highlighted the Aztecs' confidence in the avocado as an image of fruitfulness and overflow.

Notwithstanding its imagery, the avocado held down to earth incentive for the Aztecs as a supplement thick food source. It gave a significant part of their caloric admission and was a flexible fixing in their cooking. The Aztecs consumed avocados in different structures, including squashed into a spread or plunge, similar as the contemporary guacamole. Their appreciation for the organic product reached out past simple food; it became interwoven with their social and profound practices.

The appearance of Spanish travelers in the Americas in the fifteenth and sixteenth hundreds of years denoted a urgent crossroads in the avocado's set of experiences. The travelers, fascinated by the original natural products they experienced, perceived the avocado's true capacity as an important food source. The avocado advanced toward Europe, where it was developed in areas with environments helpful for its development, like Spain and Portugal. This overseas excursion denoted the start of the avocado's worldwide spread.

The avocado's spread to various landmasses reflected not exclusively its versatility as a yield yet in addition its capacity to catch the taste buds of different societies. As the natural product traversed the Atlantic and then some, it went through different changes, adjusting to the culinary inclinations of various areas. In each new objective, the avocado made some meaningful difference, turning into an image of exoticism and an esteemed expansion to neighborhood foods.

In the US, the avocado tracked down a fruitful home in California, where the Mediterranean-like environment demonstrated ideal for development. The state turned into a significant center point for avocado creation, and the Hass avocado, a cultivar with a particular pebbly skin and rich, smooth tissue, arose as a conspicuous assortment. The Hass avocado's ascent to noticeable quality during the twentieth century denoted a defining moment in the avocado's excursion, driving it from relative lack of definition to standard prominence.

The avocado's prevalence, be that as it may, confronted a brief mishap in the last 50% of the twentieth 100 years. The overall dietary patterns of the time, portrayed by an anxiety toward fats and cholesterol, cast a shadow on avocados because of their somewhat high fat substance. As low-fat eating regimens acquired favor, avocados were frequently seen with distrust, and their utilization declined.

Nonetheless, the tides started to change as dietary science advanced, testing the oversimplified thought that all fats were impeding to well-being. The acknowledgment of the differentiation among sound and undesirable fats gave another viewpoint on avocados.

The monounsaturated fats found in avocados were considered heart-sound and, combined with their variety of fundamental supplements, added to a reexamination of the organic product's dietary profile.

The late twentieth century saw a resurgence of interest in avocados, driven by changing dietary ideal models and a developing appreciation for entire, supplement thick food varieties. The avocado's excursion from being a loss from dietary patterns to a commended part of a well-being cognizant eating regimen reflected more extensive changes in buyer perspectives toward food and nourishment.

In the 21st hundred years, the avocado's notoriety took off higher than ever, filled by the ascent of health culture and online entertainment. The avocado turned into an image of current, wellbeing cognizant living, praised for its nourishing advantages and culinary flexibility. It found an especially fervent fan base among recent college grads and more youthful ages, who embraced it as a vital fixing chasing dynamic and tastefully satisfying dinners.

The avocado's social importance is maybe most distinctively depicted in its relationship with web-based entertainment, particularly stages like Instagram. The outwardly striking allure of an impeccably cut avocado or a guilefully organized avocado toast turned into a most loved subject for food bloggers, powerhouses, and home cooks the same. The hashtag #avocado turned into a virtual display, exhibiting the natural product's dynamic green tones and its bunch culinary applications.

The avocado toast pattern, which picked up speed in the mid 2010s, embodies the combination of effortlessness and complexity that describes contemporary culinary feel. The essential mix of ready avocado on toasted bread filled in as a material for culinary imagination, with lovers trying different things with a wide cluster of garnishes, from poached eggs and cherry tomatoes to radishes and microgreens. Avocado toast, past its culinary allure, turned into a social image — a symbol of a specific way of life that values wellbeing, taste, and a hint of guilty pleasure.

Avocado-driven restaurants arose in metropolitan communities, exploiting the organic product's notoriety and offering menus that exhibited its adaptability. From avocado smoothie bowls to avocado-based sweets, these foundations became shelters for those looking for a healthy and tasty feasting experience. The avocado's excursion from an unassuming natural product to a social symbol was presently finished, hardening its position in the pantheon of dearest food varieties.

However, the avocado's rising to fame isn't without its intricacies and difficulties. The flood in worldwide interest for avocados, frequently alluded to as "green gold," has prompted ecological worries, especially in locales where development is a significant industry. The ecological effect of water-escalated avocado homesteads and the related issues of deforestation for rural extension have ignited banters about the morals of avocado utilization.

Water shortage, exacerbated by environmental change, represents a critical test to avocado development. The high water necessities of avocado trees have brought up issues about the supportability of enormous scope cultivating in districts previously wrestling with water shortage. Adjusting the financial advantages of avocado creation with the need to moderate natural effect has turned into a basic thought for policymakers and partners in the business.

Deforestation connected to the extension of avocado plantations has raised worries about natural surroundings misfortune and biodiversity. As interest for avocados keeps on rising, tracking down answers for relieve these natural effects is central. Manageable cultivating rehearses, mindful obtaining, and mindfulness crusades focused on customers are all important for the continuous discourse encompassing the avocado's ecological impression.

The moral elements of avocado creation additionally stretch out to issues of fair work rehearses. In certain districts, the interest for avocados has prompted work double-dealing and unfortunate working circumstances in plantations. Tending to these worries requires an extensive methodology that considers the prosperity of both the climate and the networks engaged with avocado creation.

As shoppers become progressively aware of the social and ecological ramifications of their food decisions, the avocado business faces the test of lining up with these qualities. Endeavors to advance straightforwardness, discernibility, and supportability in the avocado store network are fundamental to guaranteeing that the organic product keeps up with its positive picture and social allure.

All in all, the avocado's excursion from old Mesoamerican civic establishments to worldwide fame is a story that entwines history, culture, and contemporary patterns. From its emblematic importance in Aztec culture to its resurgence as a superfood in the 21st hundred years, the avocado has developed because of changing culinary inclinations, dietary science, and cultural qualities.

As we enjoy the rich decency of guacamole, relish the straightforwardness of avocado toast, or investigate imaginative avocado-based dishes, perceiving the more extensive setting of the avocado's journey is fundamental. Its social significance reaches out past the domain of food; it typifies a union of custom, development, and the continuous exchange about mindful utilization in an impacting world. The avocado, with its underlying foundations immovably established ever, keeps on forming the contemporary culinary scene, making a getting through imprint on our plates and in our social awareness.

1.3 Brief exploration of health benefits

The avocado, past its culinary charm and social importance, has procured its status as a dietary force to be reckoned with, bragging a cluster medical advantages that add to generally speaking prosperity. As the world wrestles with the intricacies of current ways of life and dietary decisions, the avocado arises as a hero, offering a mix of fundamental supplements and special mixtures that help different parts of wellbeing.

One of the champion highlights of avocados is their structure of monounsaturated fats, explicitly oleic corrosive. This heart-solid fat is likewise tracked down in olive oil, and various examinations have recommended that its utilization might add to worked on cardiovascular wellbeing. Oleic corrosive has been connected to decreases in terrible cholesterol (LDL) levels while expanding great cholesterol (HDL) levels, encouraging a better lipid profile.

The monounsaturated fats in avocados are gainful for heart wellbeing as well as assume a part in supporting weight the board. Regardless of being calorie-thick, the fats in avocados add to a sensation of satiety and completion. Remembering avocados for feasts might lessen the probability of gorging and nibbling between dinners, making them a significant part of a fair and weight-cognizant eating routine.

Avocados are likewise a rich wellspring of potassium, a vital mineral engaged with keeping up with legitimate liquid equilibrium, muscle constrictions, and nerve signals. Potassium is known to balance the hypertensive impacts of sodium, possibly adding to bring down pulse levels. Sufficient potassium admission is related with a decreased gamble of stroke and cardiovascular illnesses, pursuing avocados a heart-sound decision.

Notwithstanding potassium, avocados convey a mixture of fundamental nutrients. Vitamin K, essential for blood coagulating and bone wellbeing, is bountiful in avocados. Sufficient vitamin K admission upholds bone digestion and may add to the avoidance of osteoporosis. Avocados are likewise plentiful in vitamin E, a cancer prevention agent that shields cells from harm brought about by free revolutionaries. This cell reinforcement movement might assume a part in lessening the gamble of ongoing sicknesses and advancing generally cell wellbeing.

The B-nutrient family, including B5 (pantothenic corrosive), B6 (pyridoxine), and folate (B9), is all around addressed in avocados. These nutrients are essential to different physiological cycles, including energy digestion, the development of red platelets, and the blend of synapses. Folate, specifically, is of central significance during pregnancy, as it upholds fetal turn of events and forestalls brain tube abandons.

Moreover, avocados contain a one of a kind arrangement of mixtures that add to their wellbeing advancing properties. For example, they are wealthy in lutein and zeaxanthin, two cancer prevention agents that are advantageous for eye wellbeing. These mixtures are moved in the tissues of the eyes, where they add to safeguarding against age-related macular degeneration and other eye problems.

Avocados additionally contain dissolvable and insoluble fiber, which adds to stomach related wellbeing. Dietary fiber is fundamental for keeping up with entrail routineness, forestalling clogging, and supporting a sound stomach microbiome. The blend of sound fats and fiber in avocados makes them a wonderful and stomach related well disposed expansion to dinners.

The avocado's supplement thickness and different medical advantages have prompted its consideration in different dietary methodologies, going from Mediterranean to ketogenic slims down. Its flexibility permits it to consistently coordinate into various culinary styles and inclinations, making it a significant partner for those trying to enhance their nourishment for wellbeing and essentialness.

While the medical advantages of avocados are broad, stressing the standard of dietary balance is significant. Integrating avocados into a balanced eating regimen that incorporates various supplement thick food varieties is critical to harvesting the full range of nourishing benefits. The avocado, with its one of a kind blend of sound fats, nutrients, and cell reinforcements, remains as a demonstration of the possibility that food can be both delectable and sustaining.

As the avocado keeps on earning respect for its medical advantages, logical examination into its properties and potential applications is progressing. Analysts investigate roads, for example, the effect of avocado utilization on metabolic wellbeing, its part in forestalling constant illnesses, and its consequences for different markers of prosperity. These examinations add to the developing assortment of information encompassing the avocado's multi-layered commitments to human wellbeing.

With regards to contemporary wellbeing cognizant ways of life, the avocado has turned into an image of careful eating — a decision that goes past simple taste inclinations to envelop a more extensive obligation to prosperity. The consideration of avocados in famous wellbeing patterns, for example, clean eating and plant-based counts calories, further cements their status as a go-to element for those looking for nutritious and delightful feasts.

Nonetheless, similarly as with any food, individual reactions to avocados might differ. A few people might be susceptible to avocados, encountering side effects like tingling, expanding, or trouble relaxing. It is fundamental for people with known sensitivity to practice wariness and look for clinical guidance if necessary. Also, people with explicit ailments, like pancreatitis or plastic sensitivities, may have to talk with medical services experts in regards to their avocado utilization.

Taking everything into account, the medical advantages of avocados reach out a long ways past their superb taste and culinary flexibility. Loaded with heart-solid monounsaturated fats, a variety of fundamental nutrients and minerals, and exceptional cell reinforcements, avocados offer a comprehensive bundle of supplements that help different parts of wellbeing. From cardiovascular prosperity and weight the board to eye wellbeing and processing, the avocado stands as a dietary stalwart that lines up with the standards of present day, wellbeing cognizant living. As progressing research keeps on revealing the complexities of the avocado's effect on wellbeing, its spot in the domain of superfoods is probably going to persevere, setting its standing as a flavorful and feeding partner on the excursion to prosperity.

The avocado, an organic product commended for its rich surface and flexible flavor, stretches out past its gastronomic enticement for offer a noteworthy cluster of medical advantages. As current cultures progressively focus on prosperity and careful sustenance, the avocado has arisen as a dietary force to be reckoned with, adding to heart well-being, weight the board, and by and large imperativeness.

A foundation of the avocado's wellbeing profile lies in its sythesis of monounsaturated fats, especially oleic corrosive. These heart-solid fats share similitudes with those tracked down in olive oil and are famous for their positive effect on cardiovascular wellbeing. Studies propose that the utilization of oleic corrosive might add to ideal changes in cholesterol levels, diminishing low-thickness lipoprotein (LDL) or "terrible" cholesterol while expanding high-thickness lipoprotein (HDL) or "great" cholesterol.

The monounsaturated fats in avocados, notwithstanding their calorie thickness, assume an essential part in advancing satiety and totality. Integrating avocados into feasts might assist with diminishing the probability of indulging, offering an important instrument for those looking for weight the executives. The mix of sound fats and dietary fiber in avocados makes a delightful culinary encounter that lines up with the standards of a reasonable and careful eating regimen.

Potassium, an imperative mineral, is plentiful in avocados and adds to different parts of wellbeing. Satisfactory potassium admission is related with lower pulse levels, as potassium helps balance sodium levels and loosen up vein walls. The likely decrease in hypertension risk, thusly, adds to by and large cardiovascular wellbeing, underscoring the comprehensive effect of avocados on the circulatory framework.

Notwithstanding potassium, avocados give a different scope of fundamental nutrients. Vitamin K, known for its part in blood coagulating and bone wellbeing, is available in overflow. Vitamin E, an intense cancer prevention agent, shields cells from oxidative harm brought about by free revolutionaries. The B-nutrient family, including B5 (pantothenic corrosive), B6 (pyridoxine), and folate (B9), adds to energy digestion, synapse amalgamation, and the arrangement of red platelets.

The meaning of folate in avocados turns out to be especially articulated with regards to maternal wellbeing. Folate is urgent for fetal turn of events, especially in the beginning phases of pregnancy. Satisfactory folate consumption forestalls brain tube deserts, underlining the significance of avocados as a nutritious decision for hopeful moms.

Avocados likewise gloat a one of a kind mix of cell reinforcements, including lutein and zeaxanthin, which assume a key part in supporting eye wellbeing. These mixtures are moved in the eye's tissues, where they help safeguard against age-related macular degeneration and other vision-related issues. The consideration of avocados in the eating routine adds to a thorough way to deal with visual prosperity.

The dietary fiber content in avocados further improves their commitment to stomach related wellbeing. Fiber is fundamental for keeping up with inside consistency, forestalling stoppage, and supporting a sound stomach microbiome. The cooperative connection between the sound fats, fiber, and cell reinforcements in avocados makes a profile that stretches out past basic sustenance to envelop an all encompassing effect on the body's physiological frameworks.

The avocado's supplement thickness and different medical advantages line up with different dietary methodologies, making it an important consideration in diets, for example, the Mediterranean eating routine, which underscores entire food varieties and heart-solid fats. Also, the avocado's flexibility permits it to flawlessly coordinate into ketogenic counts calories, where solid fats are focused on for energy creation.

The contemporary accentuation on careful eating and supplement thick food varieties has raised the avocado to a conspicuous situation in wellbeing society. Its part in well known dietary patterns, for example, clean eating and plant-based consumes less calories, mirrors a more extensive shift toward cognizant and purposeful food decisions. As people look for delightful and nutritious choices, the avocado stands as a characteristic partner, offering a blend of taste and medical advantages.

Logical examination keeps on disentangling the complexities of the avocado's effect on wellbeing, with studies investigating its impacts on metabolic wellbeing, irritation, and persistent illness counteraction. These examinations add to a developing collection of information that not just supports the avocado's status as a superfood yet in addition gives experiences into its expected applications in advancing in general prosperity.

While the medical advantages of avocados are significant, moving toward dietary decisions with a feeling of uniqueness and moderation is pivotal. Sensitivity to avocados, however interesting, can happen, and people with realized sensitivities ought to practice wariness and look for clinical guidance if necessary. Moreover, people with explicit ailments, like pancreatitis or plastic sensitivities, may require custom fitted direction in regards to their avocado utilization.

The avocado's joining into a balanced eating routine, portrayed by various supplement thick food varieties, is critical to enhancing its medical advantages. Its flexibility permits it to be delighted in a heap of ways — cut on toast, squashed into guacamole, mixed into smoothies, or basically eaten all alone. By embracing the avocado as a component of a different and adjusted eating design, people can outfit its full range of wellbeing advancing properties.

In the avocado's excursion from a culinary staple to a superfood is set apart by its multi-layered commitments to wellbeing. Loaded with heart-solid monounsaturated fats, fundamental nutrients, minerals, and cell reinforcements, avocados offer an all encompassing bundle of supplements. From supporting cardiovascular wellbeing and weight the executives to advancing eye wellbeing and processing, the avocado has procured its standing as a dietary force to be reckoned with. As exploration keeps on revealing the nuanced parts of its effect on wellbeing, the avocado remaining parts a flavorful and sustaining decision that rises above simple food to exemplify the standards of careful and deliberate eating.

3

Chapter 2

The Nutrient Powerhouse

The unpredictable dance of life unfurls inside the limits of the human body, a complex and remarkable orchestra of organic cycles that supports presence. At the core of this mind boggling hardware lies the basic job of supplements, those infinitesimal elements that employ the ability to direct the beat of life itself. As we dig into the significant complexities of the supplement force to be reckoned with, we set out on an excursion that crosses the domains of science, science, and nourishment, disentangling the insider facts that fuel the supernatural occurrence of human essentialness.

The groundwork of this fabulous display lies in the principal order of supplements into macronutrients and micronutrients. The macronutrients, including carbs, proteins, and fats, act as the foundation of the body's energy supply and primary trustworthiness. Carbs, in their different structures, arise as the essential wellspring of fuel, going through careful changes inside the stomach related framework to yield glucose, the phone cash of energy. Proteins, then again, stand as the draftsmen of life, taking part in the development and fix of tissues, catalysts, and chemicals. Fats, frequently insulted yet significant, add to cell layers, protection, and act as a supply of energy.

In the great woven artwork of life, micronutrients weave their mind boggling designs, unobtrusively affecting biochemical cycles and guaranteeing the consistent working of physiological hardware. Nutrients and minerals, the uncelebrated yet truly great individuals of the supplement outfit, assume essential parts in bunch natural responses. Nutrients, natural mixtures with different designs and works, capability as coenzymes or cofactors, fundamental for the synergist exercises of catalysts. Whether it be the vision-upgrading ability of vitamin A, the collagen blend represented by L-ascorbic acid, or the blood thickening coordinated by vitamin K, every nutrient arises as a particular player in the ensemble of wellbeing.

Parallelly, minerals arise as the emotionless watchmen of cell capability, with every component holding a particular key to the mind boggling locks of organic cycles. From the calcium sustaining bones and teeth to the iron arranging oxygen transport in blood, minerals act as basic parts, frequently working together with nutrients to keep up with the fragile equilibrium of homeostasis. The marriage of macronutrients and micronutrients shapes the foundation of nourishment, a unique transaction that coordinates the dance of life.

Setting out further into the profundities of this supplement odyssey, we experience the entrancing universe of cancer prevention agents. These sub-atomic superheroes stand guard against the atrocities of free extremists, unsound particles produced by metabolic cycles or natural openings. Free extremists, with their unpaired electrons, unleash devastation inside cells, prompting oxidative pressure and likely harm to cell structures. Cancer prevention agents, furnished with the capacity to kill these maverick substances, arise as the safeguards of cell uprightness, giving to them a job of principal significance in wellbeing and illness.

The complicated pathways of supplement ingestion and usage structure the nexus of metabolic speculative chemistry inside the body.

The stomach related framework, a wonder of organic designing, fills in as the door through which supplements enter the circulation system, setting out on their excursion to control cell exercises. Starches go through enzymatic changes in the mouth, stomach, and small digestive system, coming full circle in the freedom of glucose for cell energy. Proteins face the fastidious investigation of stomach related compounds, separating into amino acids that act as the structure blocks for different natural designs. Fats, going through emulsification and enzymatic cleavage, yield unsaturated fats and glycerol, indispensable for cell layers and energy stockpiling.

As the troop of supplements navigates the circulatory system, the liver stands as the cautious guardian, organizing the handling and dispersion of these imperative mixtures. Supplements, once consumed, go through changes inside the liver's chambers, guaranteeing an agreeable equilibrium in the circulation system. Abundance supplements are frequently put away for sometime later, a developmental transformation intelligent of the body's intrinsic insight to get ready for seasons of shortage.

The mind boggling dance of chemicals, organized by the endocrine framework, further refines the ensemble of supplement usage. Insulin, the maestro of glucose guideline, works with the take-up of this fundamental energy source into cells, guaranteeing a consistent stock for metabolic exercises. Glucagon, insulin's partner, prepares put away glucose when energy requests flood. The thyroid chemicals, watchmen of digestion, calibrate the speed at which cells consume energy, keeping a fragile harmony.

In the rambling scene of nourishment, the idea of bioavailability arises as an essential determinant of supplement viability. It typifies the degree and rate at which supplements are consumed and used by the body, an element impacted by different inherent and extraneous factors. The structure wherein supplements are consumed, the presence of different substances in the eating routine, and individual physiological factors on the whole add to the bioavailability of supplements, forming their effect on wellbeing.

Dietary decisions, impacted by social, financial, and individual variables, establish the groundwork for the healthful scene of people and networks. The cutting edge period observes a kaleidoscope of dietary examples, going from customary foods attached in social legacy to contemporary eating regimens formed by comfort and development. Every dietary worldview conveys its own arrangement of suggestions for wellbeing, highlighting the significance of informed decisions in molding the supplement milieu inside the body.

The persistent walk of logical request ceaselessly divulges the perplexing associations among nourishment and wellbeing, disentangling the effect of dietary examples on the gamble and movement of different sicknesses. Persistent circumstances like cardiovascular sicknesses, diabetes, and certain malignant growths display mind boggling connections to dietary propensities, featuring the critical job of sustenance as a modifiable determinant of wellbeing results. The rise of nourishing genomics, a field investigating the interchange among hereditary qualities and sustenance, further extends how we might interpret individualized reactions to dietary elements.

In the time of overflow, where the store passageways overflow with a variety of food decisions, the test lies in exploring the maze of choices to make an eating routine that orchestrates with the body's nourishing necessities. The idea of a reasonable eating regimen, frequently upheld however not generally characterized, spins around integrating different food varieties that all in all give the fundamental supplements to wellbeing. The dietary rules, molded by logical agreement, act as guides, proposing reasonable suggestions to direct people toward ideal sustenance.

The talk on nourishment rises above the domains of individual wellbeing, broadening its ringlets into worldwide worries of food security and manageability. The rising worldwide populace, combined with changing dietary examples and ecological difficulties, requires a change in outlook in the manner in which we produce, circulate, and eat food.

The many-sided interaction between horticulture, environmental change, and sustenance highlights the requirement for comprehensive methodologies that address the diverse difficulties of feeding a developing populace while saving the strength of the planet.

Inside the cauldron of nourishment research, the field of useful food varieties arises as a boondocks of investigation, offering the commitment of improved medical advantages past essential sustenance. Useful food varieties, improved with bioactive mixtures or intended to give explicit medical advantages, address a union of food science and preventive medication. From omega-3 unsaturated fat rich fish oil to probiotic-loaded yogurt, these practical food varieties make ready for a future where dietary decisions become a proactive method for advancing wellbeing and prosperity.

The social embroidery of culinary practices, a rich mosaic woven across hundreds of years, mirrors the mind boggling connection among food and character. Past its wholesome job, food fills in as a vessel for social articulation, a medium through which networks save and communicate their legacy. The customs of get-together around a common dinner, the imaginativeness of culinary methods, and the imagery implanted in conventional dishes add to the social texture that ties people and networks.

In the fantastic ensemble of life, where supplements act as the melodic notes, the idea of care in eating arises as an amicable song. Careful eating, established in the antiquated act of care, urges people to develop mindfulness and presence during the demonstration of eating. By enjoying each chomp, recognizing craving and satiety signals, and valuing the tactile experience of food, people produce a more profound association with their wholesome decisions, cultivating a reasonable and instinctive way to deal with eating.

The globalized scene of the 21st century introduces a horde of difficulties and open doors in the domain of sustenance. The approach of innovation reshapes the manner in which we access data about food, empowering people to pursue informed decisions and take part in virtual networks based on wellbeing and health. The combination of culinary practices, worked with by movement and social trade, brings about a culinary embroidery improved by different flavors and fixings.

However, in the midst of the advancement and overflow, a shadow looms — the ghost of hunger. While certain locales wrestle with the results of overnutrition and diet-related sicknesses, others bear the weight of undernutrition, where the body's fundamental supplement needs remain neglected. The worldwide test of accomplishing ideal nourishment for all requests a deliberate exertion, rising above geological limits and cultural partitions.

The talk on the supplement force to be reckoned with stretches out past the unmistakable domain of actual wellbeing, digging into the mind boggling associations among nourishment and mental prosperity.

The arising field of wholesome psychiatry investigates the effect of dietary examples on mental capability, mind-set, and psychological well-being. The stomach cerebrum hub, a bidirectional correspondence network connecting the gastrointestinal lot and the focal sensory system, turns into a point of convergence of investigation, disentangling the significant impact of stomach wellbeing on mental prosperity.

As the ensemble of life unfurls, the lifecycle of sustenance winds around its own account. From the fragile dance of supplements during pregnancy, forming the improvement of the developing hatchling, to the nuanced wholesome requirements of babies, youngsters, and teenagers, the excursion of nourishment traverses the aggregate of human life. The maturing system presents its own arrangement of contemplations, as supplement prerequisites might move, and the body's ability for retention and usage goes through inconspicuous changes.

The mind boggling dance of supplement digestion entwines with the apparition of illness, as dietary elements arise as the two heroes and adversaries in the unfurling account of wellbeing. Dietary propensities assume a vital part in the counteraction and the board of constant sicknesses, offering a modifiable road for people to impact their well-being directions. The Mediterranean eating routine, prestigious for its accentuation on organic products, vegetables, entire grains, and solid fats, remains as a signal of preventive sustenance, connected to a horde of medical advantages.

In the immense scene of nourishment, the job of dietary enhancements arises as a subject of examination and discussion. While these micronutrient definitions offer a helpful method for tending to explicit supplement lacks, their unpredictable use without clinical direction might present dangers. The mission for a panacea as enhancements frequently eclipses the nuanced interaction of supplements inside the intricate lattice of entire food varieties, stressing the significance of a comprehensive and differentiated way to deal with sustenance.

As we explore the multi-layered territory of the supplement force to be reckoned with, the apparition of falsehood and pseudoscience poses a potential threat. In a period where data multiplies at a remarkable speed, knowing the quality goods from the refuse turns into a basic expertise. Sustenance fantasies, frequently sustained by melodrama and recounted claims, highlight the requirement for a logical and proof based way to deal with dietary decisions.

The harmonious connection between actual work and sustenance adds one more layer of intricacy to the story of wellbeing. Work out, with its multi-layered benefits, impacts supplement digestion, upgrades insulin awareness, and adds to generally speaking prosperity. The sensitive balance between energy admission and consumption turns into a unique interchange, where the collaboration of nourishment and active work shapes the material of metabolic wellbeing.

In the domain of general wellbeing, nourishment arises as a foundation of preventive techniques, holding the possibility to moderate the weight of non-transferable sicknesses. Policymakers wrestle with the test of making mediations that advance solid dietary examples, address food frailty, and explore the complex trap of financial elements that impact healthful decisions. The school climate, a microcosm of society, turns into a point of convergence for nourishment training and intercessions, molding the propensities for people in the future.

The connection point among sustenance and ecological manageability frames a nexus of central significance in the 21st 100 years. The worldwide food framework, unpredictably associated with land use, water assets, and biodiversity, applies a significant effect on the strength of the planet. Reasonable farming practices, careful food creation, and dependable utilization become objectives in the journey for a tough and environmentally sound food framework.

The supplement force to be reckoned with, with its kaleidoscope of macronutrients, micronutrients, and bioactive mixtures, addresses a unique power that shapes the texture of life. As we disentangle the complexities of nourishment, we are defied with the significant acknowledgment that our dietary decisions reverberation inside the limits of our bodies as well as resound across the more extensive scenes of society and the climate. The power vested in the supplement outfit turns into a blade that cuts both ways, fit for giving essentialness and prosperity or, when employed wildly, adding to the embroidery of illness and ecological corruption.

In the great embroidery of the supplement force to be reckoned with, the story of wellbeing unfurls with every piece consumed, every supplement assimilated, and each metabolic dance arranged inside the cell domain. The orchestra of life, made by the fragile interaction of supplements, resounds with the reverberations of endless stories — accounts of strength, of sickness vanquished, and of a common excursion toward prosperity.

As we explore this many-sided scene, the basic falsehoods in disentangling the secrets of nourishment as well as in developing a significant appreciation for the job of the supplement force to be reckoned with in molding our way of living. In our decisions at the eating table, in the strategies we advocate for, and in the social stories we weave, the supplement force to be reckoned with arises as a focal hero in the legendary story of human wellbeing and prospering.

In the fabulous blend of science, culture, and individual decisions, the supplement stalwart stands as a demonstration of the noteworthy reliance between the microcosm of the human body and the cosmos of the world we possess. It entices us to step with worship, recognizing the complex dance of supplements as a great articulation of the wonder of life. As we set out on this excursion of investigation and disclosure, may we embrace the insight imbued in the supplement force to be reckoned with, remembering it as a wellspring of food as well as a significant power that shapes the material of our reality.

2.1 In-depth examination of the nutritional profile of avocados

The avocado, a verdant gem settled inside its harsh, pebbled outside, remains as a paragon of wholesome lavishness in the domain of natural products. Past its rich surface and particular flavor, the avocado is a force to be reckoned with of fundamental supplements that add to both culinary pleasure and comprehensive prosperity. As we leave on a top to bottom assessment of the nourishing profile of avocados, we disentangle the layers of nutrients, minerals, and bioactive mixtures that make this organic product a dietary mother lode.

At the center of the avocado's nourishing abundance lies its sythesis of macronutrients. Not at all like most natural products, which are overwhelmingly starches, avocados gloat a significant substance of solid fats. Most of the fat in avocados is monounsaturated fat, especially oleic corrosive — a similar heart-sound fat tracked down in olive oil. This interesting fat profile adds to the smooth surface of avocados while conferring cardiovascular advantages. Close by fats, avocados offer an unassuming measure of carbs, essentially as dietary fiber. This fiber content, containing both solvent and insoluble filaments, helps with assimilation, advances satiety, and supports in general stomach wellbeing.

Digging further into the micronutrient content, avocados arise as a rich wellspring of different nutrients and minerals. Among the nutrients, avocados are especially plentiful in vitamin K, vitamin E, L-ascorbic acid, and a few B-nutrients. Vitamin K, fundamental for blood thickening and bone wellbeing, exhibits its ability in avocados, adding to the complex trap of physiological cycles. Vitamin E, a powerful cell reinforcement, loans its defensive characteristics to avocados, safeguarding cells from oxidative harm. L-ascorbic acid, eminent for its invulnerable helping properties, adds one more layer of wholesome importance to avocados, supporting generally speaking wellbeing. The variety of B-nutrients, including B5, B6, and folate, assume fundamental parts in energy digestion, synapse combination, and DNA union, separately.

On the mineral front, avocados make a significant commitment to potassium consumption. Potassium, an imperative electrolyte, assumes a critical part in keeping up with liquid equilibrium, supporting nerve motivations, and controlling muscle constrictions. The potassium content in avocados outperforms that of bananas, a notable potassium-rich organic product. Furthermore, avocados contain essential measures of magnesium, copper, iron, and zinc, each with its own arrangement of metabolic and physiological capabilities. These minerals altogether reinforce the nourishing thickness of avocados, adding to the perplexing dance of substantial cycles.

The dietary appeal of avocados reaches out past macronutrients and micronutrients, including a troupe of bioactive mixtures with potential wellbeing advancing impacts. One such gathering of mixtures is phytosterols, plant-inferred atoms with primary similitudes to cholesterol. Phytosterols contend with cholesterol for assimilation in the gastrointestinal system, prompting diminished cholesterol retention and possibly adding to cardiovascular wellbeing.

Avocados likewise harbor carotenoids, including lutein and zeaxanthin, which are eminent for their part in eye wellbeing. These carotenoids collect in the macular area of the retina, giving security against age-related macular degeneration.

The dynamic green shade of avocados fills in as a visual demonstration of their chlorophyll content. Chlorophyll, the green color engaged with photosynthesis, has cell reinforcement properties and has been related with potential enemy of disease impacts. Moreover, avocados contain tocopherols, a gathering of mixtures having a place with the vitamin E family, further upgrading their cell reinforcement limit. The unpredictable exchange of these bioactive mixtures highlights the diverse idea of avocados as a wellspring of essential supplements as well as a useful food with potential medical advantages.

The job of avocados in cardiovascular wellbeing merits exceptional consideration, given their extraordinary fat organization. The monounsaturated fats, especially oleic corrosive, have been connected to great changes in lipid profiles, remembering decreases for low-thickness lipoprotein (LDL) cholesterol — the alleged "awful" cholesterol. The fuse of avocados into the eating routine might add to further developed lipid profiles and, thusly, a decreased gamble of cardiovascular sicknesses. Besides, the potassium content in avocados assumes a part in circulatory strain guideline, offering another cardiovascular benefit.

Avocados' true capacity in weight the executives and satiety adds one more layer to their dietary profile. In spite of their somewhat unhealthy substance, studies recommend that avocados might advance sensations of completion and decrease the longing to eat in resulting dinners. The blend of sound fats and fiber in avocados adds to delayed satiety, which might be useful for those looking for weight the executives or attempting to control calorie consumption.

The transaction among avocados and metabolic wellbeing reaches out to their effect on glucose levels. The fiber content in avocados, especially solvent fiber, dials back the processing and retention of starches, prompting a continuous arrival of glucose into the circulatory system. This can add to further developed glucose control, settling on avocados a reasonable decision for people with or in danger of type 2 diabetes.

With regards to aggravation and oxidative pressure, avocados arise as likely partners in the mission for wellbeing. The monounsaturated fats and different cell reinforcements present in avocados add to their calming properties. Persistent irritation is embroiled in the pathogenesis of different sicknesses, including cardiovascular illnesses, disease, and neurodegenerative circumstances. By relieving irritation, avocados offer a comprehensive way to deal with wellbeing support and infection counteraction.

The flexibility of avocados in culinary applications adds to their allure, making them a superb option to a wide exhibit of dishes. From guacamole, an exemplary avocado readiness, to servings of mixed greens, sandwiches, and even smoothies, avocados loan their velvety surface and rich flavor to different culinary manifestations. The culinary capability of avocados rises above flavorful dishes; they track down their direction into pastries, where their normal smoothness can be bridled to make liberal treats with a supplement thick wind.

Notwithstanding their nourishing ability, moving toward avocados as a component of a decent eating routine, taking into account individual dietary necessities and preferences is fundamental. While avocados give an overflow of restorative supplements, their calorie thickness calls for careful utilization, especially for those with explicit dietary objectives or limitations. Coordinating avocados into a shifted and adjusted diet guarantees the synergistic cooperation of supplements from various food sources, adding to in general nourishing prosperity.

The development of avocados, basically in locales with positive environments, adds to the worldwide stock of this pursued organic product. Nonetheless, the ecological impression of avocado creation, including issues like deforestation and water use in certain areas, has started discusses in regards to the supportability of avocado cultivating. As the interest for avocados keeps on rising, finding some kind of harmony between meeting purchaser inclinations and tending to ecological worries becomes basic. Manageable farming practices, combined with faithful purchaser decisions, assume a critical part in forming the future direction of avocado development.

The account of avocados unfurls past individual nourishment and culinary joy, venturing into the domain of monetary turn of events and exchange. The worldwide avocado market has seen remarkable development, powered by expanding shopper familiarity with their wholesome advantages and flexibility. Avocado-delivering nations, especially those in Latin America, have become central members in the worldwide exchange of this natural product, adding to monetary turn of events and occupations in these districts. The elements of avocado exchange highlight the complicated associations between agribusiness, business, and worldwide nourishment.

The talk on avocados addresses their nourishing credits as well as the social and social aspects implanted in their utilization. Avocados, with their starting points in Focal and South America, have turned into a worldwide peculiarity, rising above social limits and turning into a staple in different foods. The imagery of avocados reaches out past their nourishing substance; they epitomize ideas of wellbeing, extravagance, and culinary imagination. The social custom of sharing a bowl of guacamole or enjoying avocado toast mirrors the collective part of food and the social meaning of this flexible natural product.

All in all, the top to bottom assessment of the wholesome profile of avocados reveals an embroidery of energizing mixtures that position this natural product as a nourishing diamond. From heart-sound monounsaturated fats to a variety of nutrients, minerals, and bioactive mixtures, avocados offer an all encompassing mix of supplements with likely advantages for

cardiovascular wellbeing, weight the board, glucose control, and irritation. The flexibility of avocados in the culinary domain adds to their charm, making them a most loved fixing in a bunch of dishes.

As avocados climb to culinary fame, contemplations of manageability and natural effect come to the very front. Adjusting the developing worldwide interest for avocados with economical farming practices turns into a fundamental piece of the talk encompassing their creation. Customer mindfulness and decisions assume a urgent part in molding the direction of avocado development, cultivating a practical methodology that regards both the dietary lavishness of avocados and the soundness of the planet.

2.2 How avocados contribute to overall health and well-being

Avocados, past their heavenly flavor and rich surface, arise as nourishing forces to be reckoned with that fundamentally add to generally wellbeing and prosperity. This diverse natural product, known for its one of a kind blend of sound fats, nutrients, minerals, and bioactive mixtures, assumes a crucial part in supporting different parts of human wellbeing. As we dig into the complexities of how avocados add to generally speaking prosperity, we disentangle the layers of their wholesome piece and investigate the physiological advantages that make them an important option to a reasonable and empowering diet.

One of the champion elements of avocados is their noteworthy fat profile, transcendently made out of monounsaturated fats, with oleic corrosive being the essential player. Monounsaturated fats are commended for their heart-solid properties, as they have been related with enhancements in lipid profiles, especially by diminishing degrees of low-thickness lipoprotein (LDL) cholesterol — the purported "terrible" cholesterol. This one of a kind fat creation recognizes avocados from numerous different organic products, situating them as a magnificent wellspring of heart-defensive fats.

The cardiovascular advantages related with avocado utilization reach out past lipid guideline. Avocados are plentiful in potassium, a mineral significant for keeping up with sound circulatory strain levels. Potassium capabilities as an electrolyte, working with liquid equilibrium all through cells and assisting with checking the hypertensive impacts of over the top sodium consumption. The exchange between monounsaturated fats and potassium in avocados adds to their in general cardiovascular help, making them an important partner in advancing heart wellbeing.

Notwithstanding their heart-defensive characteristics, avocados are a rich wellspring of dietary fiber — a vital participant in stomach related wellbeing and generally prosperity. The fiber content in avocados, containing both dissolvable and insoluble strands, upholds gastrointestinal capability by advancing customary solid discharges, forestalling clogging, and encouraging a sound stomach microbiome. The dissolvable fiber in avocados, specifically, adds to a sensation of completion and satiety, supporting weight the board and advancing generally stomach related solace.

Avocados' job in weight the executives is highlighted by their capacity to advance satiety and diminish the longing to eat in resulting feasts. Notwithstanding their moderately fatty substance, studies propose that avocados might add to a feeling of completion, possibly prompting decreased calorie consumption over the course of the day. This satisfying impact, credited to the mix of sound fats and fiber, makes avocados a significant part of a decent eating regimen, especially for those trying to deal with their weight.

The effect of avocados on glucose levels further adds to their allure as a wellbeing advancing food. The fiber content, particularly dissolvable fiber, in avocados adds to a progressive arrival of glucose into the circulation system. This can bring about better glucose control, pursuing avocados a reasonable decision for people with or in danger of type 2 diabetes. The decent carb content, combined with the gainful fats and fiber, positions avocados as a nutritious choice for those hoping to settle their glucose levels.

The mitigating properties of avocados add to their part in supporting generally wellbeing. Persistent irritation is embroiled in the turn of events and movement of different illnesses, including cardiovascular sicknesses, malignant growth, and neurodegenerative circumstances. The monounsaturated fats and different cell reinforcements present in avocados add to their calming impacts, possibly moderating the fiery cycles inside the body. By encouraging a mitigating climate, avocados add to the general prosperity of people and may assume a part in sickness counteraction.

The rich substance of nutrients and minerals in avocados further improves their wholesome profile and their commitments to by and large wellbeing. Avocados are especially bountiful in vitamin K, which assumes an essential part in blood coagulating and bone wellbeing. Vitamin E, another strong cancer prevention agent present in avocados, shields cells from oxidative harm and supports skin wellbeing. The variety of B-nutrients, including B5, B6, and folate, add to energy digestion, synapse amalgamation, and DNA combination, separately. These nutrients, working together with the minerals like magnesium, copper, iron, and zinc tracked down in avocados, structure an exhaustive supplement group that upholds different physiological capabilities inside the body.

Avocados likewise stand apart for their substance of bioactive mixtures with potential wellbeing advancing impacts. Phytosterols, plant-determined particles with primary similitudes to cholesterol, add to the expected cardiovascular advantages of avocados by decreasing cholesterol retention in the gastrointestinal system. Carotenoids, including lutein and zeaxanthin, are related with eye wellbeing and may safeguard against age-related macular degeneration. Chlorophyll, the green shade in avocados, has cell reinforcement properties and has been connected to potential enemy of disease impacts. The complicated interaction of these bioactive mixtures adds a layer of intricacy to the wellbeing advancing properties of avocados, displaying their possible past fundamental nourishment.

The adaptability of avocados in culinary applications further upgrades their part in advancing generally wellbeing and prosperity. From the notorious guacamole to plates of mixed greens, sandwiches, and even sweets, avocados loan themselves to a different exhibit of dishes. Their velvety surface and rich flavor make them a most loved fixing in both exquisite and sweet arrangements, giving a road to integrating supplement thick choices into a differed and pleasant eating regimen.

Regardless of their horde medical advantages, moving toward avocado utilization with care, taking into account individual dietary necessities and preferences is fundamental. While avocados add to a large group of wellbeing advancing impacts, their calorie thickness calls for balance, especially for people with explicit dietary objectives or limitations. Coordinating avocados into a decent eating regimen guarantees a synergistic connection of supplements from various food sources, adding to by and large healthful prosperity.

The worldwide prevalence of avocados essentially affects agribusiness, exchange, and monetary improvement in locales where they are developed. Nations in Latin America, especially Mexico, have become central parts in the worldwide avocado market, adding to monetary development and livelihoods in these districts. The interest for avocados has flooded all around the world, driven by customer attention to their nourishing advantages and culinary flexibility. As avocados keep on being embraced as an image of refreshing eating, the financial elements of avocado creation and exchange highlight the interconnectedness of nourishment, horticulture, and worldwide business.

In the more extensive setting of food and culture, avocados rise above their dietary credits to become images of prosperity and culinary imagination. Their beginnings in Focal and South America give them social importance, yet their worldwide prevalence has made them a staple in different cooking styles. Avocado-driven dishes have become notorious images of wellbeing cognizant eating, and the social custom of sharing a bowl of guacamole or getting a charge out of avocado toast mirrors the collective part of food.

All in all, the exhaustive investigation of how avocados add to by and large wellbeing and prosperity uncovers a heap of wellbeing advancing properties that reach out a long ways past their flavorful taste. From cardiovascular help to weight the board, glucose control, calming impacts, and a rich nourishing profile, avocados arise as a flexible and important expansion to an energizing eating regimen. Their worldwide prevalence, financial effect, and social importance further highlight the complex idea of avocados, making them an image of comprehensive prosperity in the steadily developing scene of nourishment and way of life.

2.3 Exploring the impact on weight management and cardiovascular health

The mind boggling connection between dietary decisions and wellbeing results divulges a complicated transaction that reverberates across different features of prosperity. Two key spaces that attract critical consideration this talk are weight the executives and cardiovascular wellbeing. As we set out on an investigation of the effect of dietary examples on these critical parts of human wellbeing, we dig into the multi-layered collaborations between nourishment, digestion, and physiological capabilities.

Weight the executives, an enduring worry in a world wrestling with increasing heftiness rates, addresses a sensitive harmony between energy admission and consumption. The advanced way of life, portrayed by inactive ways of behaving and the wealth of energy-thick food sources, has added to the worldwide heftiness plague. Dietary examples assume a significant part in molding body weight, with the sort and amount of food sources devoured impacting the sensitive equilibrium of energy inside the body.

At the core of weight the executives lies the idea of caloric equilibrium — the connection between the calories devoured through food and refreshments and the calories used through metabolic cycles and active work. An overflow of calories prompts weight gain, while a shortage brings about weight reduction. The complex transaction of macronutrients, micronutrients, and by and large dietary organization turns into a basic consider tweaking this equilibrium and impacting weight results.

One dietary example that has acquired extensive consideration with regards to weight the board is the ketogenic diet. Described by a high fat, low sugar, and moderate protein consumption, the ketogenic diet intends to incite a condition of ketosis, where the body shifts from fundamentally involving glucose for energy to using ketones got from fat breakdown. Defenders of the ketogenic diet attest that this metabolic shift upgrades fat consuming, smothers craving, and advances weight reduction.

Research on the ketogenic diet's effect on weight the executives has yielded blended discoveries. A few investigations recommend that people following a ketogenic diet might encounter beginning weight reduction, credited to elements like decreased calorie admission and water misfortune. Nonetheless, the drawn out maintainability and potential wellbeing ramifications of the ketogenic diet remain subjects of discussion. Pundits contend that the prohibitive idea of the eating routine might prompt supplement inadequacies, and concerns affect cardiovascular wellbeing, especially with respect to raised degrees of immersed fats.

Contrastingly, plant-based consumes less calories, described by an accentuation on natural products, vegetables, entire grains, vegetables, and nuts, definitely stand out for their possible advantages in weight the board.

These weight control plans, which might incorporate varieties like vegetarianism or veganism, are many times plentiful in fiber, nutrients, minerals, and cancer prevention agents while being lower in soaked fats. The plant-based approach lines up with dietary rules advancing the utilization of supplement thick food varieties and restricting the admission of handled and unhealthy food varieties.

A few examinations propose that people sticking to plant-based diets might encounter great results in weight the board. The high fiber content of plant-based food varieties adds to satiety, advancing a sensation of completion and possibly decreasing by and large calorie consumption. Moreover, plant-based slims down are related with lower calorie thickness, making it simpler for people to devour a delightful volume of food while overseeing caloric admission. The supplement rich nature of plant-based slims down upholds generally speaking wellbeing, and their possible job in weight the board highlights the significance of dietary examples in accomplishing manageable and stimulating results.

The effect of dietary decisions on cardiovascular wellbeing addresses a basic convergence in the nexus among nourishment and prosperity. Cardiovascular illnesses, including conditions like coronary illness and stroke, stay driving reasons for worldwide bleakness and mortality. The multifaceted dance between dietary variables and cardiovascular wellbeing highlights the potential for nourishment to act as both a gamble factor and a modifiable determinant in the counteraction and the board of cardiovascular illnesses.

Immersed fats, frequently embroiled with regards to cardiovascular wellbeing, become a point of convergence in the assessment of dietary examples. These fats, normally found in creature items like meat and dairy, as well as specific tropical oils, have been related with raised degrees of low-thickness lipoprotein (LDL) cholesterol — the "awful" cholesterol. Raised LDL cholesterol is a key gamble factor for atherosclerosis, the development of plaque in veins that can prompt cardiovascular occasions.

Dietary examples that are high in immersed fats and low in other heart-solid supplements can add to an ominous lipid profile and an expanded gamble of cardiovascular sicknesses. The ketogenic diet, with its accentuation on fat admission, possibly affects cardiovascular wellbeing. While certain defenders contend that the eating routine might prompt enhancements in cardiovascular gamble factors like fatty oils and high-thickness lipoprotein (HDL) cholesterol, the height of LDL cholesterol stays a disputed matter.

Conversely, plant-based counts calories arise as promising partners in the journey for cardiovascular wellbeing. These weight control plans, wealthy in natural products, vegetables, entire grains, and nuts, give a variety of heart-sound supplements, including fiber, cell reinforcements, and unsaturated fats.

The dissolvable fiber in plant-based food sources helps lower LDL cholesterol by diminishing its assimilation in the gastrointestinal system. Moreover, cell reinforcements add to decreasing oxidative pressure and irritation, central members in the advancement of cardiovascular sicknesses.

The Mediterranean eating regimen, a very much contemplated and acclaimed dietary example, embodies the heart-solid standards of plant-based eating. Based on organic products, vegetables, entire grains, olive oil, and moderate utilization of fish and poultry, the Mediterranean eating regimen has been related with a bunch of cardiovascular advantages. Research proposes that adherence to the Mediterranean eating routine is connected to enhancements in lipid profiles, pulse, and a decreased gamble of cardiovascular occasions.

Omega-3 unsaturated fats, bountiful in greasy fish like salmon and mackerel, are essential parts of the Mediterranean eating regimen and add to its cardiovascular advantages. These fundamental unsaturated fats assume a critical part in decreasing irritation, further developing vein capability, and forestalling blood cluster arrangement. The fuse of omega-3-rich food varieties into the eating regimen lines up with proposals for cardiovascular wellbeing and highlights the capability of dietary decisions in moderating sickness risk.

The Dietary Ways to deal with Stop Hypertension (Run) diet addresses another essential dietary example that accentuates heart-quality food decisions. Intended to bring down circulatory strain, the Scramble diet energizes the utilization of organic products, vegetables, entire grains, lean proteins, and dairy items while restricting sodium consumption. The mix of supplement rich food sources and sodium limitation adds to further developed circulatory strain control and supports generally speaking cardiovascular wellbeing.

Past individual supplements and dietary examples, the idea of careful eating arises as a vital component in advancing both weight the executives and cardiovascular wellbeing. Careful eating includes developing mindfulness and presence during dinners, focusing on appetite and satiety signs, and appreciating the tangible experience of food. By encouraging a careful way to deal with eating, people can foster a better relationship with food, advancing cognizant decisions that line up with their healthful requirements and in general prosperity.

The effect of dietary decisions on weight the board and cardiovascular wellbeing reaches out past the domains of individual prosperity, impacting general wellbeing arrangements and suggestions. Public dietary rules, formed by logical agreement, assume a urgent part in illuminating people and networks about fortifying eating designs. These rules frequently underscore the significance of a decent and changed diet that incorporates a variety of supplement thick food varieties while restricting the admission of handled and unhealthy choices.

The talk on sustenance, weight the board, and cardiovascular wellbeing is innately connected to more extensive contemplations of food frameworks, horticulture, and ecological manageability. The worldwide food scene, formed by rural practices, food creation, and conveyance, impacts the accessibility and availability of energizing food decisions. The quest for practical and fair food frameworks becomes basic in guaranteeing that people and networks approach nutritious choices that help their wellbeing objectives.

The interchange between dietary examples, weight the board, and cardiovascular wellbeing is an intricate snare of connections that essentially impacts generally prosperity. In a world wrestling with the double difficulties of increasing stoutness rates and cardiovascular illnesses, understanding the nuanced connections between what we eat and what it means for our weight and heart wellbeing becomes central.

This investigation dives into the complex elements of dietary decisions with regards to weight the executives and cardiovascular prosperity, disentangling the logical experiences and commonsense ramifications that support this basic crossing point of sustenance and wellbeing.

Weight The executives: A Sensitive Equilibrium

Weight the executives is a never-ending worry in contemporary social orders where stationary ways of life and the accessibility of energy-thick food varieties add to a worldwide corpulence plague. The center rule of weight the board spins around the idea of caloric equilibrium — the balance between the calories devoured through food and refreshments and the calories used through metabolic cycles and actual work.

The cutting edge scene of dietary ways to deal with weight the executives envelops a range of procedures, each with its novel standards and implied benefits. One such dietary example that has acquired extensive consideration is the ketogenic diet. This high-fat, low-sugar, and moderate-protein approach plans to incite a condition of ketosis, where the body shifts from using glucose as its essential energy source to processing ketones got from fat breakdown.

Defenders of the ketogenic diet recommend that this metabolic shift improves fat consuming, stifles craving, and at last prompts weight reduction. Research on the momentary impacts of the ketogenic diet shows promising results, for certain examinations demonstrating beginning decreases in body weight and fat mass. Nonetheless, the drawn out supportability and potential wellbeing results of keeping a ketogenic diet remain subjects of continuous discussion inside established researchers.

Pundits express worries about the prohibitive idea of the ketogenic diet, especially its avoidance of numerous supplement thick food sources like organic products, entire grains, and certain vegetables. The potential for nourishing lacks, including insufficient admission of fundamental nutrients and minerals, brings up issues about the eating routine's general effect on wellbeing. Besides, the height of soaked fats in the eating routine, frequently through sources like red meat and high-fat dairy, prompts worries about possible ramifications for cardiovascular wellbeing.

Interestingly, plant-based eats less have arisen as a convincing and more feasible way to deal with weight the board. These dietary examples, which might incorporate vegetarianism or veganism, accentuate the utilization of plant-determined food sources like natural products, vegetables, entire grains, vegetables, and nuts, while commonly restricting or barring creature items.

A few examinations show that people sticking to plant-based diets might encounter good results in weight the executives. The high fiber content of plant-based food sources adds to sensations of completion, advancing satiety and possibly decreasing generally speaking calorie consumption. The supplement thickness of plant-based slims down permits people to eat fulfilling volumes of food while overseeing caloric admission all the more actually. The fiber-rich nature of plant-based counts calories likewise upholds stomach related wellbeing, forestalling clogging and cultivating a different and valuable stomach microbiome.

The Mediterranean eating routine, a deeply grounded and investigated dietary example, addresses a half breed approach that consolidates the standards of plant-based eating. Revolved around natural products, vegetables, entire grains, and solid fats, with moderate utilization of fish and poultry, the Mediterranean eating regimen has been related with various medical advantages, including weight the executives. The consideration of olive oil, nuts, and greasy fish gives fundamental unsaturated fats and monounsaturated fats that add to both satiety and generally prosperity.

In the domain of weight the executives, the nature of calories consumed frequently outweighs sheer amount. The idea of supplement thickness — a proportion of the fundamental supplements per calorie — becomes vital to figuring out the effect of dietary decisions. Supplement thick food varieties, plentiful in nutrients, minerals, and other bioactive mixtures, offer medical advantages past their caloric substance.

Careful eating, as a fundamental part of weight the board, accentuates developing mindfulness and presence during dinners. This training includes focusing on craving and satiety prompts, enjoying the tangible experience of food, and cultivating a better relationship with eating. By rehearsing careful eating, people can foster an increased familiarity with their dietary decisions, settling on cognizant choices that line up with their wholesome necessities and more extensive prosperity.

Cardiovascular Wellbeing: Exploring the Dietary Scene

Cardiovascular infections, enveloping circumstances, for example, coronary illness and stroke, stand as driving reasons for dreariness and mortality around the world. The perplexing connection between dietary elements and cardiovascular wellbeing highlights the potential for sustenance to act as both a gamble factor and a modifiable determinant in the counteraction and the board of cardiovascular sicknesses.

Integral to the talk on cardiovascular wellbeing is the thought of dietary fats, with a specific spotlight on immersed fats. These fats, found in creature items like meat and dairy, as well as specific tropical oils, have been customarily connected with unfriendly cardiovascular results. Raised degrees of low-thickness lipoprotein (LDL) cholesterol, frequently alluded to as the "terrible" cholesterol, are a key gamble factor for atherosclerosis — the development of plaque in corridors that can prompt cardiovascular occasions.

The ketogenic diet, portrayed by its high admission of fats, possibly affects cardiovascular wellbeing. While defenders contend that the eating routine might prompt upgrades in cardiovascular gamble factors like fatty substances and high-thickness lipoprotein (HDL) cholesterol, the rise of LDL cholesterol stays a disputed matter. The dependence on immersed fats in the ketogenic diet brings up issues about its drawn out cardiovascular ramifications, particularly given the laid out joins between soaked fats and cardiovascular illnesses.

Contrastingly, plant-based counts calories offer a heart-sound option by underscoring the utilization of unsaturated fats tracked down in nuts, seeds, avocados, and olive oil. These mono-and polyunsaturated fats have been related with further developed lipid profiles, including lower levels of LDL cholesterol and more elevated levels of HDL cholesterol. The consideration of omega-3 unsaturated fats, plentiful in greasy fish and certain plant sources like flaxseeds and pecans, further adds to cardiovascular wellbeing by lessening aggravation and supporting vein capability.

The Mediterranean eating regimen, famous for its cardiovascular advantages, lines up with these standards by integrating heart-solid fats from sources like olive oil, nuts, and greasy fish. Research proposes that adherence to the Mediterranean eating regimen is related with decreases in cardiovascular gamble factors, including further developed lipid profiles and circulatory strain control. The consideration of cell reinforcement rich food sources, like products of the soil, adds to lessening oxidative pressure and aggravation, key parts in the improvement of cardiovascular illnesses.

The Dietary Ways to deal with Stop Hypertension (Run) diet addresses one more important dietary example explicitly intended to advance cardiovascular wellbeing. Zeroed in on bringing down pulse, the Scramble diet accentuates the utilization of natural products, vegetables, entire grains, lean proteins, and dairy items, while limiting sodium admission. The synergistic blend of supplement rich food varieties and sodium limitation adds to further developed pulse control, tending to a vital part of cardiovascular prosperity.

While dietary fats assume a crucial part in cardiovascular wellbeing, different parts of dietary examples, like fiber and cell reinforcements, further add to a comprehensive way to deal with heart prosperity.

Dissolvable fiber, bountiful in natural products, vegetables, and entire grains, helps lower LDL cholesterol levels by diminishing its retention in the gastrointestinal system. Cell reinforcements, tracked down in bright leafy foods, battle oxidative pressure and irritation, offering extra layers of assurance against cardiovascular sicknesses.

Omega-3 unsaturated fats, fundamental parts of a heart-sound eating regimen, assume a huge part in diminishing cardiovascular gamble. Greasy fish, like salmon and mackerel, are rich wellsprings of these fundamental unsaturated fats. The consideration of omega-3-rich food varieties upholds generally cardiovascular wellbeing by decreasing the gamble of arrhythmias, further developing vein capability, and forestalling the arrangement of blood clusters.

The effect of dietary decisions on cardiovascular wellbeing stretches out past individual prosperity, affecting general wellbeing strategies and suggestions. Public dietary rules, molded by logical agreement, assume a critical part in illuminating people and networks about heart-good dieting designs. These rules frequently highlight the significance of a decent and changed diet that incorporates a variety of supplement thick food varieties while restricting the admission of handled and unhealthy choices.

The talk on sustenance, weight the board, and cardiovascular wellbeing is unpredictably connected to more extensive contemplations of food frameworks, horticulture, and natural supportability. The worldwide food scene, formed by agrarian practices, food creation, and conveyance, impacts the accessibility and openness of stimulating food decisions.

4

Chapter 3

Culinary Delights: Avocado in Every Bite

In the domain of gastronomy, where flavors dance and fragrances entwine, one fixing has arisen as a culinary hotshot, procuring a sought after spot on menus and in home kitchens the same. The honest green natural product, with its velvety surface and nutty connotations, has caught the hearts and taste buds of food devotees all over the planet. Enter the avocado, a flexible and nutritious joy that has turned into a staple in endless dishes, transforming conventional feasts into exceptional culinary encounters.

The excursion of the avocado's ascent to culinary fame is an entrancing one, set apart by a rich history and a mix of social impacts. Local to south-focal Mexico, the avocado, experimentally known as Persea History of the U.S, has a heredity that stretches back millennia. It was first developed by the antiquated Mesoamerican civilizations, including the Aztecs and the Maya, who worshipped it for its taste as well as for its implied medical advantages.

The's first experience with the worldwide sense of taste is a story of investigation and diverse trade. As Spanish conquerors wandered into the New World in the sixteenth hundred years, they experienced this extraordinary leafy foods it back to Europe. Throughout the long term, the avocado slowly spread to various corners of the world, adjusting to assorted environments and culinary customs.

Quick forward to the current day, and the avocado has become inseparable from contemporary food culture, embraced for its culinary adaptability and dietary profile. It's a star fixing in servings of mixed greens, spreads, and smoothies, and it even graces the plates of fancy foundations, where gourmet experts praise its unpretentious flavors and smooth surface.

One of the most notable introductions of avocado is, without a doubt, guacamole. This exemplary Mexican dish has turned into a worldwide sensation, embellishing tables at festivities and easygoing social occasions. The recipe is basic yet brilliant, requiring ready avocados, tomatoes, onions, lime juice, and a sprinkle of salt. Crushed flawlessly, guacamole typifies the substance of the avocado, offering an agreeable mix of surfaces and tastes that tempt the taste buds.

Yet, the avocado's impact reaches out a long ways past the domains of plunges and spreads. Its velvety surface makes it an optimal ally to different dishes, from sandwiches to sushi. The avocado's capacity to upgrade both the visual allure and the flavor profile of a dish deserves it a super durable spot in the culinary collection of gourmet specialists and home cooks the same.

Consider the universal avocado toast, a contemporary culinary peculiarity that has surprised the informal breakfast scene. A basic yet exquisite creation, avocado toast consolidates the rich extravagance of ready avocados with the smash of toasted bread. The expansion of different garnishes, like poached eggs, radishes, or stew chips, considers interminable inventiveness, transforming this dish into a material for culinary articulation.

The avocado's wholesome qualifications further add to its boundless approval. Wealthy in monounsaturated fats, avocados are a heart-sound decision that likewise gives fundamental nutrients and minerals. The organic product's consideration in a decent eating routine has been related with different medical advantages, including further developed cholesterol levels and improved supplement retention.

As the avocado keeps on ruling in the culinary world, gourmet experts and food lovers are investigating creative approaches to feature its adaptability. From avocado frozen yogurt to avocado chocolate mousse, the potential outcomes appear to be unfathomable. The natural product's gentle flavor fills in as a fresh start for culinary trial and error, welcoming gourmet experts to push the limits of customary recipes and investigate unforeseen pairings.

In the domain of exquisite dishes, the avocado's job reaches out past being a supporting player; it frequently becomes the overwhelming focus. Think about avocado servings of mixed greens, where cuts of ready avocado lift a basic mixture of greens into a sumptuous culinary encounter. The juxtaposition of fresh vegetables with the velvety surface of avocados makes an ensemble of flavors and surfaces that pleases the faculties.

Avocado's similarity with different cooking styles is clear in its coordination into sushi rolls. The California roll, a well known sushi variation, highlights avocado close by crab or impersonation crab, cucumber, and ocean growth. The smooth consistency of the avocado gives a superb differentiation to different fixings, adding a layer of complexity to the sushi experience.

Past the flavorful domain, avocados consistently progress into the area of treats. Avocado-based desserts have built up momentum for their remarkable blend of extravagance and wholesome advantages. Avocado chocolate mousse, for example, has turned into a #1 among wellbeing cognizant treat lovers. The smooth surface of ready avocados, when mixed with cocoa powder and improved to taste, makes a debauched treat that rivals customary chocolate mousse.

The avocado's culinary excursion likewise converges with the developing interest for plant-based and veggie lover choices. As individuals embrace plant-driven eats less, the avocado stands apart as a flexible and fulfilling substitute for dairy and creature fats. It tends to be stirred into a rich dressing, fill in for spread in heated products, or basically delighted in as a fantastic and sustaining nibble.

In the realm of drinks, avocados show up. Avocado smoothies, frequently joined with natural products like banana and berries, offer an invigorating and nutritious option in contrast to conventional natural product smoothies. The avocado's unobtrusive flavor adds profundity and richness, changing a basic beverage into a wonderful dinner substitution or post-exercise boost.

The worldwide ubiquity of avocados has changed culinary scenes as well as influenced agrarian practices. As interest for avocados has flooded, especially in North America and Europe, locales with reasonable environments have seen an expansion in avocado development. This has not been without challenges, as worries about water utilization, deforestation, and fair work rehearses in avocado-creating districts have come to the front.

The avocado's excursion from a nearby delicacy in Mexico to a worldwide sensation has not been without debate. The avocado business has confronted examination for its natural and social effect, with discusses encompassing issues like deforestation, water shortage, and fair work rehearses. As shopper mindfulness develops, there is a call for additional maintainable and moral practices inside the avocado production network.

Notwithstanding these difficulties, the avocado remaining parts an image of culinary development and social combination. Its flexibility to different cooking styles, its healthful advantages, and its capacity to lift both basic and complex dishes have gotten its place as a dearest fixing in kitchens around the world. From road food slows down to Michelin-featured cafés, the avocado keeps on molding culinary patterns and move gourmet experts to push the limits of innovativeness.

The avocado's impact reaches out past the bounds of conventional recipes, motivating culinary specialists and home cooks to explore different avenues regarding surprising pairings and strong flavor mixes. Avocado mixed drinks, for instance, have turned into a stylish decision for those looking for a remarkable and invigorating beverage. The rich surface of avocados can be integrated into refreshments like margaritas or smoothies, adding a delectable quality that improves the general drinking experience.

As the culinary world keeps on developing, so does the avocado's part in molding the manner in which we see and experience food. Its excursion from a territorial specialty to a worldwide sensation reflects the more extensive patterns in contemporary cooking, where variety, manageability, and development become the overwhelming focus. The avocado's story is one of versatility and variation, as it meshes its direction into the texture of culinary practices across societies and landmasses.

3.1 Creative and delicious avocado recipes

The avocado, with its tasty surface and gentle, rich flavor, plays rose above its part as a simple fixing to turn into a culinary sensation. Past the darling avocado toast and exemplary guacamole, inventive culinary experts and home cooks are investigating the tremendous capability of this flexible natural product, presenting a heap of innovative and heavenly recipes that grandstand its novel characteristics.

We should start with breakfast, where the avocado can offer a striking and nutritious expression. Avocado and egg breakfast bowls have acquired fame for their straightforwardness and healthy goodness. Picture a completely ready avocado half supporting a prepared egg, sprinkled with spices and flavors. The outcome is an agreeable marriage of smooth avocado and runny egg yolk, making a morning meal dish that is both outwardly engaging and fulfilling.

For those with a sweet tooth, avocado finds its direction into breakfast smoothie bowls and parfaits. Mixed with natural products like banana, berries, and a sprinkle of almond milk, avocado includes a smooth surface. Layered with granola and finished off with coconut pieces or nuts, these avocado-imbued breakfast treats are a brilliant method for beginning the day on a healthy note.

Continuing on toward lunch, the avocado's adaptability sparkles in plates of mixed greens that go past the normal. An avocado and dark bean salad joins velvety avocado lumps with good dark beans, corn, tomatoes, and a fiery lime dressing. The outcome is a reviving and supplement pressed salad that can remain solitary as a light lunch or act as a dynamic side dish.

Avocado additionally takes the spotlight in grain bowls, where it very well may be matched with quinoa, earthy colored rice, or farro. Envision a bowl loaded up with a bright variety of simmered vegetables, avocado cuts, and a shower of cilantro-lime dressing.

The avocado's lavishness supplements the nuttiness of the grains, making a wonderful and healthy dinner that takes care of both taste and nourishment.

For an innovative bend on conventional sandwiches, think about the avocado BLT. This variety of the exemplary bacon, lettuce, and tomato sandwich presents rich avocado cuts, raising the flavor profile and adding a sumptuous touch. The blend of firm bacon, succulent tomatoes, new lettuce, and smooth avocado makes an ensemble of surfaces and tastes that makes certain to satisfy the sense of taste.

Avocado's culinary ability stretches out to warm dishes too. Avocado pasta, a dish that has acquired prevalence as of late, highlights a rich avocado sauce mixed with garlic, basil, and Parmesan cheddar. Thrown with still somewhat firm pasta, this dish offers a wanton and tasty option in contrast to customary pasta sauces. The avocado sauce covers the pasta strands, making a lavish and fulfilling dinner.

In the domain of hors d'oeuvres, avocado is a headliner in imaginative and swarm satisfying dishes. Avocado fries, for instance, take the idea of conventional fries to another level. Cuts of avocado are covered in breadcrumbs and prepared or broiled to brilliant flawlessness. The outcome is a firm outside giving way to a rich inside, making these avocado fries an overpowering and better option in contrast to potato fries.

Avocado likewise transforms sushi rolls past the universal California roll. The fiery fish and avocado roll, for example, joins the smoothness of avocado with the intensity of hot fish, making an enticing flavor mix. The expansion of cucumber and a sprinkle of fiery mayo finishes the group, bringing about a sushi roll that is however outwardly engaging as it could be delightful.

For an invigorating and surprising tidbit, avocado gazpacho gives a cutting edge contort on the conventional Spanish virus soup. Mixing ready avocados with cucumber, chime peppers, tomatoes, and a sprinkle of garlic, this chilled soup offers an eruption of flavors and a smooth surface. Decorated with new spices or a dab of Greek yogurt, avocado gazpacho is a magnificent method for whetting the hunger.

The avocado's excursion into the domain of fundamental courses go on with dishes that feature its versatility and capacity to improve different flavor profiles. Avocado and lime barbecued chicken, for instance, includes a marinade of crushed avocado, lime juice, and cilantro. The chicken, when barbecued flawlessly, flaunts a smoky flavor with a smidgen of citrus, supplemented by the rich avocado marinade.

For a plant-based principal course, avocado enchiladas give a fantastic and tasty choice. Loaded down with a combination of dark beans, corn, and diced avocado, the enchiladas are covered in a lively green enchilada sauce produced using mixed avocados, tomatillos, and

green chilies. Prepared to effervescent flawlessness, these avocado enchiladas are a delectable turn on an exemplary Mexican dish.

In the realm of barbecuing, avocados can be changed into a flavorful enjoyment with barbecued avocado parts. The intensity of the barbecue upgrades the normal smoothness of the avocado, making a smoky flavor that matches well with different fixings. Barbecued avocados can be loaded up with fixings like salsa, quinoa, or barbecued shrimp, offering a flexible material for culinary imagination.

For a combination of flavors, consider avocado and mango salsa-bested fish tacos. The blend of flaky fish, sweet mango, and rich avocado salsa makes an ensemble of flavors and surfaces. Enveloped by warm tortillas and embellished with cilantro and a press of lime, these fish tacos offer a tropical and fulfilling feasting experience.

Yet again as the day advances into dessert, avocados demonstrate their flexibility. Avocado chocolate truffles are a debauched and virtuous treat that joins ready avocados with dull chocolate, cocoa powder, and a hint of pleasantness. The outcome is a rich and velvety truffle that melts in the mouth, offering a great end to any feast.

Avocado likewise finds its direction into the domain of frozen treats with avocado frozen yogurt. Mixed with coconut milk and improved to taste, avocado frozen yogurt conveys a smooth surface and an unpretentious avocado flavor. Whether delighted in a cone, as a parfait, or close by a warm pastry, avocado frozen yogurt adds a reviving and extraordinary curve to the universe of frozen treats.

For the individuals who lean toward a no-heat choice, avocado lime cheesecake gives a smooth and citrus-imbued dessert experience. The avocado adds to the cheesecake's satiny surface, while lime juice adds a lively and invigorating note. Set on a graham saltine outside layer and chilled flawlessly, this avocado lime cheesecake is a brilliant method for covering off a dinner.

As we dive into the domain of refreshments, avocado keeps on leaving an imprint with its presence in smoothies, mixed drinks, and even espresso. Avocado smoothies, frequently mixed with organic products like banana, pineapple, and spinach, offer a sustaining and empowering drink that is however fulfilling as it very well might be nutritious.

In the realm of mixed drinks, the avocado margarita has acquired ubiquity for its exceptional bend on the exemplary Mexican beverage. Mixed with ready avocados, tequila, triple sec, and lime squeeze, this mixed drink conveys a velvety and tasty involvement in a smidgen of refinement. Embellished with a cut of avocado or a salted edge, the avocado margarita is an invigorating and startling drink.

For espresso lovers, avocado espresso gives a smooth and sans dairy option in contrast to customary flavors. Mixing ready avocados with fermented espresso brings about a foamy and smooth refreshment. Improved with a dash of honey or agave syrup, avocado espresso offers a rich and fulfilling choice for those looking for a novel turn on their day to day caffeine fix.

The culinary scene of avocado reaches out past individual recipes to envelop more extensive subjects of maintainability and moral obtaining. As the interest for avocados keeps on rising around the world, worries about ecological effect, fair work rehearses, and dependable cultivating rehearses have come to the front.

Avocado cultivating, especially in districts like Mexico and portions of South America, has confronted examination for its possible commitment to deforestation, water shortage, and social issues. As buyers become more aware of the starting points of their food, there is a developing development towards supporting manageable and morally obtained avocados.

All in all, the imaginative and tasty universe of avocado recipes is a demonstration of the natural product's unmatched flexibility and allure. From breakfast to dessert, avocados flawlessly incorporate into a wide cluster of dishes, adding a smooth surface, an unobtrusive flavor, and a large group of nourishing advantages. As gourmet experts and home cooks keep on trying different things with inventive approaches to exhibit this cherished organic product, the avocado's excursion from a straightforward fixing to a culinary star is set to develop and rouse for quite a long time into the future.

3.2 Avocado's role in enhancing taste and texture in various dishes

The avocado, with its rich surface and gentle, rich flavor, has turned into a culinary wonder, praised for its capacity to raise taste and surface in a bunch of dishes. From canapés to treats, this flexible organic product has woven its direction into the texture of contemporary cooking, contributing not exclusively unmistakable taste yet in addition a one of a kind richness improves the general feasting experience.

How about we start with hors d'oeuvres, where the avocado becomes the overwhelming focus in imaginative and tasty dishes. Avocado bruschetta, for instance, changes the exemplary Italian tidbit into a velvety pleasure. Ready avocado cuts are layered on toasted bread and finished off with a combination of diced tomatoes, red onions, garlic, and basil. The outcome is an agreeable mix of surfaces, with the velvety avocado filling in as the ideal foil to the energetic and tart tomato blend.

Continuing on toward soups, the avocado's capacity to improve taste and surface is displayed in avocado soup varieties. A chilled avocado and cucumber soup, for example, consolidates the cooling properties of cucumber with the smoothness of avocado, making an invigorating and smooth soup. Mixed with yogurt, lime juice, and a sprinkle of jalapeño for an unobtrusive kick, this soup is a demonstration of the avocado's flexibility in both flavor and consistency.

Mixed greens, a material for culinary imagination, offer sufficient chances for the avocado to sparkle. An avocado and grapefruit salad, for example, weds the rich lavishness of avocado with the succulent pleasantness of grapefruit fragments. Prepared with blended greens, sugar coated nuts, and a citrus vinaigrette, this salad not just tempts the taste buds with differentiating flavors yet in addition delights with a mix of rich and fresh surfaces.

In the domain of primary courses, the avocado's job stretches out past being a simple garnish; it frequently turns into an essential part that changes the dish. Think about barbecued chicken with avocado salsa, where impeccably barbecued chicken bosoms are embellished with an energetic salsa produced using diced avocado, tomatoes, red onions, cilantro, and lime juice. The avocado salsa not just adds an explosion of variety to the plate yet additionally presents a rich component that supplements the barbecued chicken delightfully.

Avocado's presence in pasta dishes is no less effective. Avocado pesto pasta, a contemporary curve on customary pesto, integrates ready avocados into the sauce. Mixed with basil, garlic, pine nuts, Parmesan cheddar, and olive oil, the avocado adds to a richly smooth pesto that covers the pasta strands. The outcome is a pasta dish that weds the lavishness of avocado with the striking kinds of exemplary pesto.

For a fish charm, avocado matches consistently with ceviche. Avocado shrimp ceviche, for instance, joins the briny decency of shrimp with the rich surface of diced avocados. Marinated in lime juice, cilantro, and red onions, the ceviche accomplishes an ideal equilibrium of flavors, with the avocado adding a smooth touch to each nibble.

Presented with tortilla chips or on fresh tostadas, this dish is a festival of differentiating tastes and surfaces.

In the realm of sandwiches, wraps, and burgers, avocados have turned into a darling element for their capacity to upgrade both flavor and mouthfeel. Take, for example, the exemplary turkey and avocado club sandwich. The rich cuts of avocado, settled between layers of turkey, bacon, lettuce, and tomato, hoist the sandwich from customary to exceptional. The avocado's smoothness goes about as a characteristic sauce, adding to the general succulence and fulfillment of each chomp.

Veggie lover and vegetarian dishes, as well, benefit from the avocado's capacity to give a wonderful richness. Avocado and dark bean tacos, for instance, offer a plant-put together elective that doesn't think twice about respect to flavor or surface. Crushed avocado fills in as a delightful base, giving a smooth differentiation to the generous dark beans and the mash of new vegetables. Finished off with salsa and a sprinkle of lime crema, these tacos feature the avocado's flexibility in vegan cooking.

As we adventure into the domain of side dishes, cooked vegetables with avocado crema offer a delightful blend of broiled goodness and smooth guilty pleasure. Vegetables like yams, Brussels fledglings, and cauliflower, cooked to caramelized flawlessness, are joined by a dab of avocado crema. The crema, made by mixing avocados with lime juice, garlic, and yogurt, adds a rich and cooling component to the warm broiled vegetables.

Avocado's part in upgrading taste and surface expands consistently into the domain of worldwide cooking. In sushi, the avocado's rich consistency adds a layer of refinement to rolls and nigiri. The avocado and salmon roll, for example, joins the rich lavishness of avocado with the smooth surface of new salmon. The outcome is a sushi roll that not just enjoyments the sense of taste with a sensitive interchange of flavors yet additionally presents a lavish, rich surface.

In Mexican cooking, guacamole is the famous portrayal of avocado's capacity to upgrade taste and surface. Pounded avocados are mixed with tomatoes, onions, cilantro, lime juice, and a sprinkle of salt to make this dearest plunge. Whether gathered up with tortilla chips or utilized as a garnish for tacos and nachos, guacamole is a festival of the avocado's capacity to contribute a smooth and tasty component to different dishes.

The avocado's excursion into the culinary world isn't restricted to flavorful dishes; it flawlessly changes into the domain of sweets, where its novel characteristics add profundity and lavishness. Avocado chocolate mousse, a #1 among wellbeing cognizant pastry lovers, replaces customary dairy with ready avocados. Mixed with cocoa powder, sugar, and a sprinkle of vanilla concentrate, the outcome is a smooth chocolate mousse that is however liberal as it seems to be righteous.

For a tropical turn, avocado tracks down its direction into key lime pie. Avocado key lime pie, with its rich avocado filling and rich graham wafer hull, offers a reviving interpretation of the exemplary sweet. The avocado adds to the pie's lavish surface, while the key lime flavor adds a lively kick. Finished off with whipped cream or a dab of avocado-imbued yogurt, this treat is a demonstration of the natural product's flexibility in the domain of desserts.

In the realm of frozen treats, avocado frozen yogurt has arisen as a well known decision for those looking for a sans dairy elective. Mixed with coconut milk, improved to taste, and beat to smooth flawlessness, avocado frozen yogurt offers a brilliant and invigorating treat choice. Whether delighted in a cone, matched with new natural product, or showered with chocolate sauce, avocado frozen yogurt features the natural product's capacity to carry a rich smoothness to frozen delights.

Drinks, as well, are not invulnerable to the avocado's impact on taste and surface. Avocado smoothies, frequently mixed with organic products like banana, mango, and spinach, make a plush and fulfilling drink.

The avocado's gentle flavor permits it to flawlessly coordinate into an assortment of smoothie mixes, adding a rich consistency that upgrades the general drinking experience.

Mixed drinks, with their unending potential for imagination, greet the avocado wholeheartedly. The avocado margarita, a contemporary wind on the exemplary Mexican beverage, highlights mixed avocados with tequila, triple sec, and lime juice. The outcome is a smooth and tasty mixed drink that weds the extravagance of avocado with the citrusy kick of a margarita. Embellished with a cut of avocado or a salted edge, this mixed drink is a festival of the natural product's capacity to hoist drinks.

As we praise the avocado's job in upgrading taste and surface across different dishes, recognizing the more extensive ramifications of its popularity is significant. The worldwide interest for avocados has prompted worries about ecological manageability, fair work rehearses, and dependable cultivating. In districts where avocados are developed, issues like deforestation, water utilization, and social effect have gone under examination.

Endeavors to advance feasible and moral avocado cultivating rehearses are getting forward movement, with drives zeroing in on dependable obtaining, water preservation, and local area commitment. As shoppers become more aware of the beginnings of their food, there is a developing development towards supporting avocado makers who focus on ecological stewardship and social obligation.

All in all, the avocado's job in upgrading taste and surface is a demonstration of its flexibility and boundless allure in the culinary world. From starters to pastries, the avocado flawlessly incorporates into various dishes, contributing a smooth surface and a gentle flavor that improves the general feasting experience. As gourmet specialists and home cooks keep on investigating imaginative approaches to exhibit the avocado, its excursion from a straightforward organic product to a culinary symbol is set to develop and motivate into the indefinite future.

3.3 Tips for incorporating avocados into different cuisines

Avocados, with their smooth surface and gentle flavor, have turned into a worldwide culinary sensation, rising above lines and foods. Their flexibility permits them to flawlessly incorporate into various dishes, from customary Mexican passage to contemporary worldwide food. In this investigation of ways to integrate avocados into various culinary customs, we dive into the craft of culinary combination, commending the avocado's capacity to upgrade and hoist flavors across the globe.

Mexican Food:

In their local land, avocados are a fundamental piece of Mexican cooking, and dominating their utilization in customary dishes is a culinary experience. Guacamole, the famous avocado plunge, is a staple.

To raise its flavor, pick ready avocados, squash them to your ideal consistency, and afterward add finely cleaved onions, tomatoes, cilantro, lime juice, and a spot of salt. For an additional kick, add diced jalapeños or a hint of hot sauce. The key is tracking down the right harmony among smoothness and surface.

Tacos, a cherished Mexican road food, give one more material to avocado inventiveness. Consider finishing off your tacos with cuts of ready avocado or crushing them to make a smooth and tasty taco spread. The cool, velvety surface of the avocado wonderfully supplements the strong kinds of prepared meats, beans, and new salsa.

Asian Combination:

Avocados consistently coordinate into different Asian cooking styles, giving a one of a kind wind to customary dishes. Sushi, with its fragile flavors and surfaces, invites the expansion of avocado. Avocado rolls, frequently including rice, ocean growth, and new vegetables, give a fantastic difference to the exquisite notes of soy sauce and wasabi. For a more debauched encounter, attempt the combination of avocado with fiery fish in sushi rolls.

In Thai cooking, avocados can be integrated into servings of mixed greens for a smooth component. A green papaya salad with avocado joins the freshness of destroyed papaya with the perfection of ready avocados, making an agreeable mix of surfaces. The dressing, ordinarily highlighting lime juice, fish sauce, and stew, integrates the flavors in a wonderful way.

Mediterranean Style:

The Mediterranean eating regimen, known for its accentuation on new produce and solid fats, tracks down an ideal partner in avocados.

For a Mediterranean-roused salad, consolidate diced avocados with tomatoes, cucumbers, olives, and feta cheddar. Shower with olive oil and sprinkle with oregano for a reviving and nutritious dish.

Avocado hummus is a superb combination of Mediterranean and avocado flavors. Just mix ready avocados with chickpeas, garlic, tahini, and lemon juice to make a velvety hummus variety. Serve it with pita bread or new vegetables for a fantastic and supplement pressed plunge.

Southwestern Joys:

In Southwestern cooking, where strong flavors and generous fixings rule, avocados sparkle in dishes like avocado and dark bean plates of mixed greens. Consolidate diced avocados with dark beans, corn, red onions, and chime peppers. The rich avocado fills in as a lavish partner to the powerful kinds of the beans and the pleasantness of the corn.

For a Southwestern interpretation of burgers, think about garnish your patties with cuts of smooth avocado. The coolness of the avocado adjusts the intensity from flavors or jalapeños, making a burger experience that is both fulfilling and tasty.

European Tastefulness:

Indeed, even in the refined universe of European cooking, avocados have tracked down a spot. In Italian dishes, avocado coordinates well with the effortlessness of bruschetta. Top toasted bread with a combination of diced avocados, tomatoes, garlic, and basil for a wonderful hors d'oeuvre that consolidates velvety and crunchy surfaces.

For a sumptuous pasta experience, integrate avocados into a velvety Alfredo sauce. Mix ready avocados with garlic, Parmesan cheddar, and a sprinkle of lemon juice. Throw the sauce with fettuccine or linguine for a pasta dish that is both debauched and shockingly light.

Center Eastern Enchantment:

In Center Eastern cooking, avocados carry a rich component to dishes like shawarma. Top your shawarma wraps with cuts of ready avocado to add an invigorating and smooth surface that supplements the strong kinds of flavored meats and tahini sauce.

For a cutting edge contort on conventional plunges like baba ganoush, consider integrating avocados. Mix simmered eggplant with ready avocados, garlic, tahini, and lemon juice for a smooth and delightful plunge. This combination of surfaces and flavors makes a remarkable variety that matches well with pita bread or new vegetables.

African Motivations:

In African cooking, avocados can upgrade both flavorful and sweet dishes. For an exquisite choice, integrate avocados into a couscous salad. Join cooked couscous with diced avocados, cherry tomatoes, cucumbers, and a shower of lemon vinaigrette for a light and invigorating dish.

In treats, avocados can assume an astounding part. Avocado chocolate mousse, with its smooth surface and rich flavor, can be imbued with African flavors like cardamom or cinnamon for an additional layer of intricacy.

Indian Combination:

In Indian cooking, where flavors and aromatics become the dominant focal point, avocados can be integrated into both customary and combination dishes. Avocado raita, an invigorating yogurt-based side dish, consolidates diced avocados with yogurt, mint, and cumin for a cooling backup to hot curries.

For a cutting edge curve on samosas, think about filling the baked good with a combination of flavored potatoes, peas, and crushed avocados. The richness of the avocado adds a magnificent component to the conventional flavorful filling.

Caribbean Pleasures:

In the dynamic and delightful universe of Caribbean food, avocados add a dash of smoothness to dishes like jerk chicken. Top your jerk chicken with cuts of ready avocado to adjust the intensity of the flavors with a cool and smooth surface.

For a tropical and invigorating beverage, think about an avocado and pineapple smoothie. Mix ready avocados with pineapple, coconut milk, and a sprinkle of lime juice for a smooth and outlandish drink that catches the pith of the Caribbean.

Ways to integrate Avocados Across Foods:

Pick Ready Avocados: The way to integrating avocados effectively is picking ready ones. Search for avocados that yield somewhat to delicate strain and have a velvety surface.

Try different things with Surfaces: Avocados can be pounded, cut, diced, or mixed, offering various surfaces. Try different things with various arrangements to find what suits your dish best.

Match with Reciprocal Flavors: Avocados taste gentle that matches well with various fixings. Try different things with integral flavors like citrus, spices, flavors, and differentiating surfaces to make an even dish.

Think about Temperature: Avocados can be appreciated in both warm and cold dishes. While they add a smooth surface to warm pasta dishes, they likewise carry a reviving component to chilled plates of mixed greens or sushi rolls.

Investigate Sweet and Appetizing Blends: Don't restrict avocados to exquisite dishes. Investigate their flexibility in sweet deals with like pastries, smoothies, and shakes. The smooth surface of avocados can add a sumptuous quality to sweet dishes.

Utilize Avocado as a Solid Fat Substitute: Avocados can be a nutritious substitute for fixings like margarine, cream, or mayonnaise in specific recipes. Supplant these fixings with squashed avocados for a better turn.

Try different things with Worldwide Flavors: Avocados act as an unbiased material, making them ideal for exploring different avenues regarding worldwide flavors. Have a go at integrating flavors and spices from various foods to make one of a kind flavor profiles.

Balance Flavors: Whether you're adding avocados to a hot Mexican dish or a gentle European serving of mixed greens, take a stab at balance. The smooth surface of avocados can assist with relaxing strong flavors or add wealth to milder dishes.

Remember the Lime: The exemplary mix of avocados and lime upgrades the natural product's flavor and forestalls searing. A crush of lime juice adds a citrusy punch as well as helps save the dynamic green shade of avocados.

Show Matters: Avocados add to the flavor as well as upgrade the visual allure of a dish. Consider various approaches to introducing avocados, whether cut conveniently on top or pounded and integrated into the dish.

As culinary limits keep on obscuring, the joining of avocados into different cooking styles is a demonstration of the natural product's widespread allure. From the roads of Mexico to the kitchens of Europe and the lively business sectors of Asia, avocados have procured their place as a culinary chameleon, adjusting to and improving the kinds of each and every culture they experience. As you set out on your avocado culinary excursion, let innovativeness be your aide, and enjoy the wonderful subtleties this adaptable natural product brings to your table.

Avocados, with their smooth surface and gentle, rich flavor, have risen above their local starting points to turn into a worldwide culinary peculiarity. From the sun-soaked fields of Mexico to kitchens all over the planet, avocados have found a spot in a variety of foods, every variation mirroring the extraordinary qualities and inclinations of the way of life they experience. As we set out on an investigation of how avocados flawlessly coordinate into different culinary practices, we disentangle the flexible ways this cherished organic product enhances the woven artwork of worldwide flavors.

Mexican Culinary Authority:

In the heartland of avocado development, Mexico, this green pearl isn't simply a fixing; it's a social symbol. At the center of Mexican cooking is guacamole, a basic yet impeccable mix of crushed avocados, tomatoes, onions, cilantro, lime juice, and a smidgen of salt. This quintessential avocado dish features the natural product's capacity to converge with strong flavors, making an amicable ensemble that upgrades the conventional tortilla chip insight.

Avocado's impact reaches out past guacamole in Mexican culinary practices. Tacos, a road food #1, welcome the rich expansion of cut avocados. Whether it's barbecued meats, fiery salsas, or exquisite beans, the avocado's cool and smooth surface gives a reviving contradiction to the strong and lively kinds of Mexican road passage.

Asian Combination Twists:

Avocado's process toward the east leads it into the core of Asian food, where it consistently incorporates into different culinary scenes. Sushi, a cunning marriage of flavors and surfaces, embraces avocados in rolls and nigiri. Avocado rolls, loaded up with rice, ocean growth, and a collection of new vegetables, offer a smooth and rich difference to the sensitive kinds of crude fish.

In Thai food, avocados add a tropical touch to plates of mixed greens. A combination of surfaces arises in a green papaya and avocado plate of mixed greens, joining the freshness of destroyed papaya with the rich non-abrasiveness of ready avocados.

The dressing, an energetic blend of lime juice, fish sauce, and bean stew, integrates the sweet and flavorful notes, making a reviving plate of mixed greens with a touch of smoothness.

Mediterranean Mixture:

The avocado, a newbie to the Mediterranean storeroom, tracks down its place in plates of mixed greens and plunges, adding a sumptuous touch to the district's healthy charge. A Greek plate of mixed greens takes on a rich turn with the expansion of ready avocado cuts, supplementing the briny olives, feta cheddar, and succulent tomatoes. The marriage of surfaces lifts the plate of mixed greens into a fantastic and nutritious dish.

Avocado hummus, a combination of Center Eastern and avocado flavors, consolidates the wealth of chickpeas with the rich surface of avocados. Mixed with garlic, tahini, and a sprinkle of lemon squeeze, this plunge offers a wonderful option in contrast to customary hummus. Presented with pita bread or new vegetables, avocado hummus carries a smooth polish to the mezze table.

Southwestern Ensemble:

In the sun-kissed scenes of the American Southwest, avocados flawlessly coordinate into the energetic and strong kinds of the locale. Mixed greens burst with variety and newness as avocados wed with dark beans, corn, and hot salsas. The rich avocado fills in as a cooling specialist against the intensity of bean stew peppers, making a wonderful exchange of flavors.

Southwestern burgers take on a connoisseur bend with the expansion of cut avocados. The cool and smooth surface of the organic product supplements the smoky kinds of barbecued meats, changing an exemplary burger into a culinary encounter that is both liberal and invigorating.

European Style Embraces Avocado:

The avocado, once extraordinary, has turned into a sweetheart of European kitchens, adding a bit of extravagance to exemplary dishes. Bruschetta, an Italian appetizer staple, takes on a smooth persona when finished off with diced avocados, tomatoes, and new basil. The avocado's rich wealth supplements the firmness of the toasted bread, making a magnificent starter.

In French cooking, the avocado fits current understandings of exemplary recipes. A niçoise salad, commonly highlighting fish, eggs, and olives, gains a rich redesign with the expansion of avocado cuts. The outcome is a plate of mixed greens that orchestrates the strong kinds of the Mediterranean with the rich smoothness of avocados.

Center Eastern Sorcery:

Avocados show up in Center Eastern dishes, contributing a smooth touch to conventional flavors. Shawarma, a cherished road food, tracks down a cool and rich friend in cut avocados.

Settled in wraps or served on platters, avocados give a mitigating differentiation to the flavored meats and tart tahini.

A cutting edge curve on baba ganoush includes mixing simmered eggplants with avocados, making a sleek plunge that joins the smokiness of eggplant with the richness of avocados. Presented with warm pita bread, this combination plunge carries a rich component to the Center Eastern table.

African Motivations:

In the immense and different culinary scenes of Africa, avocados track down their direction into plates of mixed greens, stews, and even treats. A couscous salad, famous in North Africa, takes on a rich note with the expansion of diced avocados. Matched with sweet-smelling flavors, new spices, and a shower of olive oil, this salad turns into a festival of differentiating surfaces and flavors.

In pastries, avocados can be changed into awesome treats. Avocado and coconut milk frozen yogurt, injected with tropical flavors, offers a reviving decision to a hot African dinner. The avocado's rich consistency mixes flawlessly with coconut milk, making a sans dairy treat that is both liberal and healthy.

Indian Developments:

In the energetic embroidery of Indian cooking, avocados add a smooth component to conventional dishes. Avocado raita, a cooling yogurt-based side dish, consolidates diced avocados with yogurt, mint, and cumin. This invigorating backup supplements hot curries, biryanis, and kebabs, furnishing an explosion of coolness with each spoonful.

A cutting edge turn on samosas includes filling the cake pockets with a combination of flavored potatoes, peas, and crushed avocados. The avocado's smoothness turns into an amazing component in the conventional flavorful filling, making a combination tidbit that spans the culinary practices of India and the West.

Caribbean Charms:

In the tropical heaven of the Caribbean, avocados add a dash of extravagance to both exquisite and sweet dishes. Jerk chicken, with its red hot flavors, tracks down a smooth accomplice in cut avocados. The smooth surface of avocados tempers the intensity of the jerk preparing, making a reasonable and tasty dish.

For a reviving drink, think about an avocado and pineapple smoothie. Mixing ready avocados with sweet pineapple and a sprinkle of coconut milk brings about a rich and extraordinary beverage that catches the quintessence of the Caribbean. Served over ice, this smoothie turns into a magnificent taste of tropical heaven.

Ways to dominate Avocado Incorporation:

Choosing the Ideal Avocado: The excursion starts with picking the right avocados. Search for organic products that yield marginally to delicate tension, demonstrating readiness. Be aware of the variety, with an energetic green tone flagging ideal preparation.

Dominating Surface Varieties: Avocados loan themselves to different surfaces - cut, diced, squashed, or mixed. Explore different avenues regarding various arrangements to accomplish the ideal consistency for your dish.

Matching with Reciprocal Flavors: Avocados have a gentle flavor that matches well with a variety of fixings. Try different things with reciprocal flavors like citrus, spices, flavors, and surfaces to make an agreeable dish.

Taking into account Temperature Elements: Avocados nimbly explore both warm and cold dishes. While their velvety surface supplements warm pasta dishes, it likewise adds an invigorating component to chilled plates of mixed greens or sushi rolls.

Investigating the Sweet and Flavorful Range: Avocados aren't restricted to appetizing dishes; their adaptability stretches out to sweet deals with like pastries, smoothies, and shakes. Embrace the rich surface to add an extravagant quality to your sweet manifestations.

Avocado as a Sound Fat Substitute: Avocados can act as a nutritious substitute for fixings like spread, cream, or mayonnaise. Supplant these parts with squashed avocados to give a better wind to your recipes.

Worldwide Flavoring Experiences: Avocados go about as an unbiased material for trial and error with worldwide flavors. Integrate flavors and spices from various cooking styles to make remarkable and unforeseen flavor profiles.

Finding Some kind of harmony of Flavors: Whether acquainting avocados with a hot Mexican dish or a gentle European serving of mixed greens, hold back nothing. The smooth surface of avocados can either smooth striking flavors or add extravagance to gentler dishes.

Remember the Lime: The exemplary mix of avocados and lime improves the organic product's flavor as well as forestalls sautéing. A crush of lime juice adds a citrusy punch and jam the dynamic green shade of avocados.

Consideration regarding Show: Avocados contribute not exclusively to the taste yet in addition to the visual allure of a dish. Consider various approaches to introducing avocados - whether flawlessly cut on top or squashed and integrated into the dish.

As culinary limits keep on obscuring, avocados arise as an image of solidarity in variety, consistently adjusting to and improving the worldwide sense of taste. From the enthusiastic roads of Mexico to the exquisite tables of Europe and the zest loaded kitchens of India, avocados demonstrate that great taste knows no boundaries. Thus, as you leave on your culinary excursion with avocados, let your inventiveness stream, and enjoy the wonderful subtleties this adaptable organic product brings to your table.

5

Chapter 4

A Taste of Avocado Wisdom

In the curious town of Serenica, settled in the midst of moving slopes and rich plantations, there existed an exceptional peculiarity known as the Avocado Celebration. This yearly festival was not simply a social occasion of local people to enjoy the rich green organic product; it was an otherworldly encounter that unfurled like an embroidery of intelligence, winding around together the strings of custom, culture, and a smidgen of the magical.

As day break broke upon the arrival of the celebration, the air was pregnant with expectation. Locals clamored through the restricted cobblestone roads, their giggling and babble reverberating through the enchanting houses enhanced with lively bougainvillea. The celebration grounds, a rambling knoll lined by old oak trees, anticipated the party that would before long result.

At the core of Serenica stood the venerated Avocado Woods, a hallowed space where the avocado trees, their branches weighty with organic product, held court. Legend had it that these trees were implanted with old insight, and the people who participated in the celebration would be conceded a sample of this heavenly understanding.

The celebration initiated with a stylized parade drove by the town seniors. Wearing streaming robes enhanced with avocado themes, they conveyed a brilliant platter bearing the principal avocado of the time. This emblematic organic product, known as the "Insight Avocado," was said to hold onto the pith of edification.

As the older folks moved toward the Avocado Forest, a quiet fell over the group. The sun cast a warm shine upon the get-together, and a feeling of veneration settled among the members. The main senior, a respected figure with a streaming white facial hair growth, raised the Insight Avocado high, offering a quiet supplication to the spirits of the woods.

The natural product was then painstakingly cut open, uncovering its energetic green tissue. The fragrance floated through the air, an olfactory introduction to the banquet that would follow. The principal cut was ceremoniously proposed to the most seasoned resident, a centenarian named Elena, who professed to have gone to each Avocado Celebration since youth.

Elena's eyes shone with a blend of wistfulness and expectation as she relished the smooth nibble. An aggregate breath held by the spectators was delivered in a murmur of help and satisfaction when Elena broke into a wide grin. The Insight Avocado had spoken, and its message was one of assertion and progression.

With the formal opening total, the celebration changed into a kaleidoscope of varieties, sounds, and flavors. Slows down lined the knoll, offering a variety of avocado-implanted luxuries. From avocado frozen yogurt to barbecued avocado sticks, the inventiveness of the town culinary specialists exceeded all logical limitations.

Among the merriments, one slow down stuck out — the Astute Avocado Prophet. Monitored by a baffling figure known as the Prophet Attendant, this stall offered customized readings in light of the examples tracked down in cut avocados. Members would introduce their picked avocados, and the Prophet Manager would decipher the plan of the organic product's tissue to disclose experiences into their lives.

Sofia, a youthful craftsman with dreams as immense as the Serenica sky, moved toward the Savvy Avocado Prophet with a blend of interest and suspicion. She painstakingly chose an avocado and gave it to the Prophet Guardian, who capably cut it open with a formal blade. The example that arose appeared to hit the dance floor with deeper implications.

The Prophet Manager, clad in a shroud enhanced with avocado-molded runes, concentrated on the avocado's tissue with a power that verged on the supernatural. After a snapshot of quietness that felt like an unending length of time, the Prophet Manager talked. "Sofia, your creative undertakings will prove to be fruitful past creative mind. Embrace the obscure, for inside it lies the material of your predetermination."

Sofia left the Shrewd Avocado Prophet with a newly discovered feeling of direction. The celebration, she understood, was a festival of a dearest organic product as well as a course for the indication of dreams. Serenica, with its Avocado Celebration, was a safe house where the normal rose above into the unprecedented.

As the sun plunged beneath the skyline, projecting shades of pink and gold across the sky, the celebration took on an otherworldly quality. The Avocado Woods, presently washed in the delicate gleam of lights, turned into the focal point of collective narrating. Townspeople accumulated around, their countenances enlightened by the warm light, as elderly folks told stories of the otherworldly beginnings of the Avocado Celebration.

As per the old legend, Serenica was established by a meandering clan looking for a land favored by the divine beings. Legend held that the divine beings, in a token of heavenly fortune, gifted the clan with avocado seeds, educating them to sow the seeds and construct their town around the sacrosanct trees. The Avocado Woods, subsequently, turned into the core of Serenica — a living demonstration of the town's cooperative relationship with nature.

Captivated by the legends, a gathering of youthful locals set out on an evening time journey to the core of the Avocado Forest. Directed by the delicate sparkle of fireflies, they explored the twisted ways between the antiquated trees. The air was thick with the powerful scent of ready avocados, and the stir of leaves conveyed murmurs of ages past.

As the gathering arrived at the focal point of the woods, they found a clearing where a giant avocado tree, its branches going after the sky, remained as a quiet sentinel. The storage compartment bore perplexing carvings portraying scenes from the town's set of experiences, a visual narrative of the heavenly association among Serenica and the avocado.

Enchanted by the sight, the gathering felt an extraordinary presence encompassing them. Maybe the spirits of the forest had stirred, welcoming the locals to cooperative with the insight imbued in the actual quintessence of the trees. As one, the gathering shut their eyes and expanded their hands, as though looking for a material association with the insight that lay lethargic inside the old woods.

At that time, an aggregate vision unfurled — an embroidery of recollections, dreams, and the interconnected accounts of Serenica's occupants. The Avocado Forest, it appeared, was not just a vault of information but rather a living substance that reflected the shared perspective of the town.

Back in the celebration glade, the party went on into the evening. The air resonated with chuckling, music, and the clunking of glasses loaded up with avocado-imbued drinks. The Shrewd Avocado Prophet, presently encompassed by a crowd of enthusiastic members, kept on revealing the secrets hid inside the examples of cut avocados.

In the mean time, a gathering of locals accumulated around a huge fire, passing around guitars and sharing tunes that reverberated through the slopes. The gleaming blazes cast moving shadows on the essences of the locals, their eyes mirroring the fellowship brought into the world of shared customs and the aggregate insight of the Avocado Celebration.

Among the revelers, Miguel, a carefully prepared rancher with endured hands and a heart receptive to the mood of the land, stood examining the flashing flares. He had been going to the celebration as far back as he could recall, yet every year brought a recharged feeling of miracle.

For Miguel, the Avocado Celebration was in excess of a festival; it was a fellowship with the patterns of nature, a sign of the interconnectedness between the earth and its stewards. As he tasted on some avocado-implanted tea, the glow spread through him, establishing him right now.

In a fortunate development, Miguel wound up in discussion with Isabella, a botanist who had as of late shown up in Serenica to concentrate on the novel characteristics of the town's avocado trees. Interested by Miguel's profound association with the land, Isabella listened eagerly as he divided his experiences into the cooperative relationship among the townspeople and the Avocado Woods.

"Miguel," Isabella said, her eyes shimmering with interest, "there's an unprecedented thing about the avocados in Serenica. The structure of their tissue, the wealth of their flavor — it's not normal for anything I've experienced in my examination. Do you trust there's a logical clarification for the uniqueness of these avocados?"

Miguel contemplated Isabella's inquiry, his look floating towards the Avocado Woods somewhere far off. "There's a sorcery in this land, Isabella. It's not just about the dirt or the environment; it's about the narratives woven into the underlying foundations of these trees. The avocados here convey the aggregate insight of ages."

As the night wore on, the celebration arrived at its crescendo. An excellent huge fire was lit in the focal point of the knoll, and residents assembled around for the finishing service — a custom dance went down through the ages. The dance, known as the "Avocado Three step dance," was a smooth articulation of appreciation for the plentiful gather and a representative token of solidarity.

Under the twilight sky, the locals moved in synchrony, their strides repeating the heartbeat of the earth. The dance was a demonstration of the recurrent idea of life, where each step addressed a season, each whirl a snapshot of change. As the music twirled around them, the locals felt a significant association with the rhythms of the normal world.

Among the artists, Sofia and Miguel wound up accomplices in the Avocado Three step dance. Their developments streamed flawlessly, as though directed by an inconspicuous power. At that time of shared concordance, Sofia felt a profound reverberation with the heartbeat of Serenica, while Miguel detected the progression of custom flowing through their dance.

As the Avocado Three step dance arrived at its decision, the residents assembled in a circle around the huge fire, their countenances enlightened by the warm gleam. The central senior ventured forward, holding a crate loaded up with avocado seeds. Every resident, youthful and old, took a seed and made a quiet wish prior to establishing it in the sacrosanct soil of the celebration grounds.

The demonstration of sowing avocado seeds represented the coherence of life, the death of astuteness starting with one age then onto the next. The Avocado Forest, with its old trees and enchanted quality, took the stand concerning this immortal custom — an embroidery of trust woven into the texture of Serenica's presence.

As the principal light of day break painted the skyline, flagging the finish of the celebration, the locals assembled briefly of reflection. The Avocado Forest, washed in the delicate tones of morning, remained as a quiet gatekeeper, its branches weighed down with the commitment of future harvests.

The celebration had come to a nearby, however its embodiment waited in the hearts of the locals. The flavor of avocado insight, bestowed through the customs, stories, and shared encounters, would keep on forming the predetermination of Serenica. In the hug of custom and the murmurs of the Avocado Woods, the town tracked down an immortal wellspring of motivation — a sample of shrewdness that rose above the limits of existence.

4.1 Connecting mindfulness and nutrition

In the cutting edge embroidery of wellbeing and prosperity, the strings of care and nourishment are complicatedly woven, framing an amicable example that rises above simple actual food. The excursion towards all encompassing wellbeing includes not just feeding the body with the right supplements yet in addition developing a careful consciousness of the whole eating experience. This combination of care and sustenance welcomes people to set out on an extraordinary investigation of their relationship with food, opening a significant comprehension of the interconnectedness between psyche, body, and sustenance.

At the core of this coordination lies the idea of careful eating — a training established in care, which empowers an uplifted consciousness of the current second without judgment. Careful eating stretches out past the demonstration of devouring food; it includes the whole range of eating, from the determination of fixings to the enthusiasm for flavors, surfaces, and the physiological prompts of craving and satiety.

The excursion into careful eating frequently starts with an interruption — a cognizant snapshot of reflection before the principal chomp. In a world portrayed by speedy ways of life and in a hurry utilization, this respite fills in as an extraordinary demonstration, a recovery of the ceremonial idea of eating. It prompts people to consider what they are eating as well as why and how they are devouring their food.

Think about a straightforward demonstration: the stripping of an orange. In a careful eating setting, this apparently unremarkable undertaking changes into a sensorial encounter. The surface of the orange strip under fingertips, the eruption of citrus fragrance as the skin is penetrated, and the cadenced movement of stripping become a fountain of vibes that anchor the psyche to the present. With each sense drew in, the demonstration of eating turns into a multisensory venture, encouraging a significant association with the food being devoured.

Careful eating isn't tied in with forcing unbending guidelines or limitations; rather, it is an encouragement to enjoy the wealth of the current second. It urges people to pay attention to their bodies, perceiving the unobtrusive signs of yearning and completion. This increased mindfulness enables people to settle on informed decisions in view of their exceptional healthful necessities, encouraging a reasonable and natural way to deal with eating.

In the domain of careful sustenance, the idea of the "mind-stomach association" arises as a vital point of convergence. The stomach, frequently alluded to as the "second mind," houses an intricate organization of neurons that speak with the focal sensory system. This complex transaction between the brain and the stomach impacts stomach related processes as well as profound prosperity.

Consider a situation where an individual consumes a feast hurriedly, diverted by outside upgrades, for example, work messages or web-based entertainment warnings. In this surged express, the body's pressure reaction might be enacted, prompting poor assimilation and supplement retention. Running against the norm, moving toward a feast with care and a casual perspective establishes a climate helpful for ideal processing.

Besides, the brain stomach association reaches out past the actual domain, affecting close to home states and mental prosperity. Stress and nervousness, whenever left neglected, can appear as stomach related uneasiness and effect the body's capacity to acclimatize supplements. On the other hand, careful eating goes about as an ointment for the brain, encouraging a feeling of quiet and presence that decidedly impacts the stomach related process.

As people set out on the excursion of interfacing care and nourishment, the job of appreciation arises as a core value. Developing appreciation for the food on one's plate and the complex cycles that carried it to completion ingrains a significant feeling of appreciation.

From the ranchers who kept an eye on the yields to the hands that pre-arranged the feast, every part of the food venture turns into a string in the embroidery of interconnectedness.

The act of offering thanks for food reaches out past its wholesome substance; it envelops the social, natural, and social components of sustenance. In a globalized existence where food frequently navigates huge distances to arrive at the plate, careful eaters foster an intense consciousness of the natural impression related with their dietary decisions. This mindfulness fills in as an impetus for feasible and cognizant food utilization, cultivating an association with the more extensive biological system.

Chasing careful nourishment, the idea of "eating the rainbow" arises as an energetic and outwardly convincing rule. The different cluster of varieties present in products of the soil mirrors a range of phytonutrients, each offering remarkable medical advantages. From the cell reinforcement rich purple tints of berries to the beta-carotene-stuffed orange tones of carrots, devouring different beautiful food sources turns into a festival of nourishing variety.

Past the wholesome advantages, the demonstration of enjoying a rainbow of food varieties lines up with the standards of care, empowering people to draw in with the visual, olfactory, and gustatory components of their feasts. Each chomp turns into an investigation of flavors and surfaces, cultivating a tangible wealth that rises above the utilitarian demonstration of sustenance.

A careful way to deal with sustenance likewise includes embracing the idea of instinctive eating — an attunement to the body's normal signals and rhythms. In this present reality where outside prompts, for example, carbohydrate levels and piece measures frequently direct dietary decisions, natural eating urges people to entrust their bodies and develop a humane relationship with food.

The natural eating structure contains standards like regarding yearning and totality, dismissing the eating routine mindset, and looking for fulfillment in eating. By tuning into the body's signs of craving and satiety, people can cultivate a fair and maintainable way to deal with sustenance. This attunement to interior signals advances a feeling of organization and independence, freeing people from outer food rules and cultivating a good connection with their bodies.

With regards to careful nourishment, the act of "eating with goal" arises as a core value. This deliberate methodology includes adjusting one's dietary decisions to individual qualities, wellbeing objectives, and moral contemplations. Whether driven by a longing to help neighborhood ranchers, lessen natural effect, or address explicit wellbeing concerns, eating with goal turns into a cognizant demonstration that rises above flashing desires.

Careful nourishment likewise welcomes people to investigate the idea of "careful cooking." The readiness of feasts, frequently saw as a task in the rushed speed of current life, turns into a chance for imaginative articulation and taking care of oneself. Taking part during the time spent choosing new fixings, cleaving vegetables with care, and injecting dishes with purposeful flavors changes cooking into a thoughtful practice.

The demonstration of careful cooking reaches out past the person to envelop collective and social aspects. Sharing a home-prepared dinner turns into a token of association, a method for feeding the body as well as the securities that structure the texture of local area. In the common experience of planning and participating in a dinner, people fashion associations that rise above the value-based nature of eating.

In the crossing point of care and sustenance, the act of careful tasting arises as a pondering investigation of refreshments. Past the practical part of hydration, careful tasting includes enjoying each taste with mindfulness, whether it be some natural tea, a newly prepared espresso, or a reviving smoothie. The demonstration of careful tasting stretches out past the gustatory experience to embrace the tangible subtleties of temperature, smell, and surface.

As people explore the scene of careful nourishment, the idea of "careful guilty pleasure" turns into a nuanced investigation of the relationship with treats and liberal food varieties. In a culture frequently portrayed by dichotomous reasoning around "great" and "terrible" food sources, careful extravagance supports a fair and non-prohibitive methodology. It includes relishing treats with goal, savoring the tangible experience, and developing a virtuous pleasure in extraordinary treats.

In the domain of careful sustenance, the idea of "careful development" entwines with the actual component of prosperity. The body, saw as a basic piece of the psyche body association, benefits from development rehearses that encourage a feeling of presence and encapsulation. Whether through yoga, careful strolling, or different types of deliberate development, people develop an agreeable connection among body and psyche.

The combination of care and sustenance stretches out to the act of "careful sustenance arranging." This deliberate methodology includes arranging feasts with mindfulness, taking into account dietary requirements, flavor inclinations, and the delight got from the demonstration of eating. Careful sustenance arranging rises above inflexible dinner plans, offering an adaptable structure that adjusts to the steadily changing scene of individual requirements and inclinations.

As people embrace the standards of careful sustenance, they become sensitive to the interconnectedness of their prosperity with more extensive cultural and natural settings. The demonstration of careful eating turns into an impetus for cognizant buyer decisions, motivating people to help moral and supportable food rehearses. This far reaching influence stretches out past private prosperity to add to the aggregate prosperity of the planet.

In the junction of care and sustenance, the act of "careful assimilation" arises as a pensive investigation of the physiological cycles engaged with separating and absorbing supplements. Past the unthinking perspective on processing, careful assimilation includes tuning into the body's signs, perceiving the transaction among craving and fulfillment, and encouraging an appreciation for the sustenance got.

The excursion of associating care and sustenance stretches out to the job of "careful quietness" in encouraging a thoughtful space for eating. In a culture where feasts are many times joined by outer upgrades, for example, TV or electronic gadgets, the act of careful quiet includes relishing each chomp with centered consideration. This deliberate quietness makes a safe-haven for the faculties, permitting people to draw in with the tactile experience of eating completely.

In the consistently developing scene of careful sustenance, the idea of "careful variation" turns into a core value. This versatile methodology includes recognizing that individual nourishing necessities shift in light of elements, for example, age, action levels, and medical issue. Careful variation welcomes people to develop an adaptable and responsive relationship with their bodies, changing healthful decisions in view of the powerful idea of prosperity.

As people cross the way of interfacing care and sustenance, the idea of "careful reflection" arises as a groundbreaking practice. This intelligent investigation includes occasionally stopping to survey one's relationship with food, distinguishing designs, and recognizing the developing idea of dietary requirements. Careful reflection turns into a compass that guides people towards a more profound comprehension of the unpredictable interaction between brain, body, and sustenance.

In the embroidery of careful nourishment, the act of "careful coordination" turns into a consistent converging of care standards with day to day existence. Past being an assigned practice, care incorporates into the texture of regular activities, impacting dietary decisions, cooking ceremonies, and the enthusiasm for sustenance. Careful coordination fills in as an extension that interfaces the thoughtful domain of care with the unique embroidery of day to day presence.

As people explore the scene of careful sustenance, the idea of "careful strength" arises as a sustaining force. This strong methodology includes recognizing that the excursion towards all encompassing wellbeing might experience difficulties, misfortunes, and vacillations. Careful strength welcomes people to develop a humane relationship with themselves, perceiving that prosperity is a dynamic and advancing interaction.

In the convergence of care and nourishment, the excursion turns into a consistent investigation — a powerful dance between the thoughtful domains of care and the unmistakable components of sustenance. This interconnected methodology rises above the limits of a prescriptive dietary model, offering an adaptable and individualized structure that adjusts to the steadily changing scene of prosperity.

All in all, the blend of care and sustenance discloses an embroidery of interconnectedness — a lively transaction between brain, body, and sustenance. The excursion towards comprehensive wellbeing includes the utilization of supplements as well as a careful familiarity with the whole eating experience. Through practices like careful eating, appreciation, and instinctive sustenance, people leave on a groundbreaking investigation that rises above the limits of traditional dietary standards. In this rich embroidery, each string addresses a feature of prosperity, adding to an all encompassing and agreeable relationship with food and self.

4.2 The joy of savoring each bite mindfully

In the whirlwind of present day life, where time appears to get past us like sand, the basic demonstration of enjoying each nibble carefully arises as a significant practice — a door to a more extravagant and seriously satisfying relationship with food. Past the utilitarian capability of sustenance, careful eating welcomes people to draw in with the tactile woven artwork of flavors, surfaces, and fragrances that unfurl with every piece. It is an excursion into the current second, a thoughtful investigation that rises above the rushed speed of everyday presence.

At the center of careful eating is the development of mindfulness — a cognizant presence that changes the demonstration of eating into a multisensory experience. As people leave on this excursion, they are urged to offer their complete focus of real value, saving interruptions and tuning into the orchestra of vibes that go with each nibble.

Think about a straightforward dinner — a slyly pre-arranged dish with dynamic tones, a captivating smell, and a mixture of surfaces. In the domain of careful eating, this turns out to be something other than food; it changes into a blowout for the faculties. The initial step is to stop — a snapshot of tranquility before the principal chomp. This interruption isn't just an actual discontinuance however a psychological progress, a conscious shift into a condition of uplifted mindfulness.

In this purposeful delay, people are welcome to notice the visual show of the dinner — the transaction of varieties, the course of action of fixings, and the imaginative articulation of the culinary specialty. This visual blowout turns into a preface to the gustatory experience, making way for a careful commitment with the demonstration of eating.

The excursion into careful eating then reaches out to the olfactory domain — a tangible investigation of the fragrances that float from the plate. The feeling of smell, unpredictably connected to the feeling of taste, fills in as an aide into the universe of flavors anticipating disclosure. Each breathe in turns into a preface to the gastronomic experience, elevating the expectation and arousing the sense of taste.

As the primary piece meets the tongue, the material element of careful eating becomes an integral factor. The surfaces of the food — fresh, smooth, crunchy, or delicate — welcome people to investigate the actual impressions that go with each nibble.

The demonstration of biting, frequently consigned to the foundation in rushed dinners, turns into a point of convergence, a cognizant commitment with the mechanical and tactile parts of the eating system.

Careful eating isn't tied in with complying with a bunch of rules or limitations; rather, it is a challenge to draw in with food in a way that sustains both the body and the soul. The training urges people to enjoy the extravagance of flavors, appreciate the supporting characteristics of fixings, and develop a significant appreciation for the overflow that supports them.

In the hurrying around of present day life, where dinners are many times consumed in a hurry or before screens, the act of careful eating turns into an extreme demonstration of disobedience — a recovering of the ceremonial idea of sustenance. It welcomes people to make a holy space for feasts, liberated from the interruption of outer interruptions, and to move toward each nibble with a feeling of veneration.

As people drench themselves in the craft of careful eating, they find that the training goes past the limits of the feasting table — it penetrates the whole range of the food venture. From the determination of fixings to the planning of dinners, care turns into a core value, implanting each step with goal and presence.

Consider the demonstration of shopping for food through a careful focal point. In this thoughtful methodology, people draw in with the most common way of choosing new produce with a feeling of interest and wisdom. The dynamic shades of leafy foods become a visual exhibition as well as an impression of the wholesome variety that is standing by.

Careful shopping for food stretches out to a consciousness of the beginning of food — the excursion it has embraced from ranch to table. This natural care encourages an association with the more extensive biological system, inciting people to think about the ecological effect of their food decisions and to help reasonable and moral practices.

The act of careful eating likewise welcomes people to investigate the idea of "careful cooking." In the domain of culinary creation, every fixing turns into a range of flavors ready to be blended. The demonstration of slashing vegetables, estimating flavors, and mixing a stewing pot turns into a thoughtful practice — a chance for inventive articulation and taking care of oneself.

The planning of dinners, frequently saw as an unremarkable task in the surge of day to day existence, changes into a sacrosanct demonstration with regards to careful cooking. It includes drawing in with the cycle with a feeling of presence, mixing the fixings with goal, and relishing the catalytic change that happens in the pot of the kitchen.

As the smell of a home-prepared dinner penetrates the air, careful cooking stretches out its impact to the common and social elements of sustenance. Sharing a dinner arranged with careful consideration turns into a token of association — a method for sustaining the body as well as the securities that structure the texture of local area.

In the domain of careful eating, the idea of "eating with every one of the faculties" turns into a core value. This tactile commitment goes past the ordinary comprehension of taste and contact to incorporate the full range of human insight. From the visual allure of a dish to the hear-able joy of a fresh nibble, careful eating turns into a festival of the lavishness of tangible experience.

The coordination of care into the demonstration of eating additionally includes an investigation of the "mind-stomach association." This unpredictable interchange between the psyche and the stomach impacts stomach related processes as well as profound prosperity. The act of careful eating fills in as a scaffold that associates the mental and physiological elements of sustenance.

Consider a situation where an individual consumes a dinner in a surged and occupied state. The body's pressure reaction might be actuated, affecting stomach related processes and compromising the assimilation of supplements. In actuality, moving toward a dinner with care and a casual perspective establishes a climate helpful for ideal processing.

The brain stomach association reaches out past the actual domain to impact profound states. Stress and nervousness, whenever left ignored, can appear as stomach related distress and effect the body's capacity to absorb supplements. Careful eating goes about as a relieving demulcent for the brain, encouraging a feeling of quiet and presence that decidedly impacts the stomach related process.

In the investigation of careful eating, the idea of "careful dividing" arises as a pondering way to deal with serving and devouring food. In a culture where piece sizes are in many cases directed by outer standards, careful distributing urges people to adjust to their own craving and completion signs. It includes serving and consuming amounts that line up with the body's one of a kind necessities, encouraging a reasonable and instinctive way to deal with sustenance.

Careful parceling likewise includes an investigation of the idea of "careful guilty pleasure." In a world frequently described by dichotomous reasoning around "great" and "terrible" food varieties, careful extravagance welcomes people to move toward treats and liberal food varieties with mindfulness and expectation. It includes enjoying these exceptional treats without culpability, completely captivating with the tangible joy they offer.

The act of careful eating stretches out its impact to the idea of "careful hydration." Past the practical part of extinguishing thirst, careful hydration includes enjoying each taste with expectation and mindfulness.

Whether it be some natural tea, a reviving glass of water, or a restoring smoothie, the demonstration of careful tasting turns into a scrutinizing investigation of refreshments.

In the crossing point of care and nourishment, the idea of "careful transformation" turns into a core value. This versatile methodology includes perceiving that individual wholesome necessities change in view of elements, for example, age, action levels, and ailments. Careful transformation welcomes people to develop an adaptable and responsive relationship with their bodies, changing healthful decisions in view of the powerful idea of prosperity.

As people cross the scene of careful eating, the idea of "careful reflection" turns into an extraordinary practice. This intelligent investigation includes occasionally stopping to survey one's relationship with food, distinguishing designs, and recognizing the advancing idea of wholesome requirements. Careful reflection turns into a compass that guides people towards a more profound comprehension of the complicated interchange between brain, body, and sustenance.

The union of care and sustenance welcomes people to embrace the idea of "careful mix." This incorporation includes meshing care standards into the texture of day to day existence, impacting dietary decisions as well as cooking ceremonies, supper time rehearses, and the enthusiasm for sustenance. Careful mix turns into an extension that interfaces the thoughtful domain of care with the unique embroidery of day to day presence.

In the domain of careful eating, the act of "careful quietness" arises as a pensive investigation of the physiological cycles engaged with separating and absorbing supplements. In a culture where dinners are many times joined by outer improvements, for example, TV or electronic gadgets, the act of careful quiet includes enjoying each nibble with centered consideration. This purposeful quiet makes a safe-haven for the faculties, permitting people to draw in with the tangible experience of eating completely.

The excursion of interfacing care and sustenance stretches out past the person to envelop cultural and ecological aspects. Careful eating turns into an impetus for cognizant customer decisions, motivating people to help moral and economical food rehearses. This expanding influence reaches out past private prosperity to add to the aggregate prosperity of the planet.

In the consistently developing scene of careful sustenance, the idea of "careful flexibility" arises as a sustaining force. This versatile methodology includes recognizing that the excursion towards all encompassing wellbeing might experience difficulties, misfortunes, and variances. Careful strength welcomes people to develop a humane relationship with themselves, perceiving that prosperity is a dynamic and advancing cycle.

In the embroidery of careful nourishment, the delight of enjoying each chomp carefully turns into a festival of the current second. It is an encouragement to dial back, to draw in with the tactile wealth of food, and to cultivate a significant association with the demonstration of eating. In this scrutinizing investigation, each nibble turns into a snapshot of euphoria — a passage to a more supported and satisfying life.

4.3 Cultivating a healthy relationship with food through avocado wisdom

In the domain of sustenance and prosperity, the avocado stands as an image of healthy sustenance and the encapsulation of an all encompassing way to deal with wellbeing. Developing a sound connection with food through "avocado insight" goes past the simple utilization of a supplement rich natural product; it digs into the standards of careful eating, appreciation, and reasonable sustenance. This investigation unfurls as an embroidery, winding around together the wholesome advantages of avocados with the careful practices that go with their utilization.

Avocado insight, at its center, welcomes people to move toward food with a feeling of care — a cognizant mindfulness that rises above the rushed speed of present day life. Careful eating, with regards to avocado insight, includes relishing each chomp with aim and presence. The avocado, with its velvety surface and rich flavor, turns into a vessel for a tactile excursion that stretches out past the demonstration of sustenance.

Think about the basic demonstration of cutting into a ready avocado. The blade coasts through the smooth skin, uncovering the lively green tissue inside. In the domain of avocado insight, this second turns into a pondering encounter — an acknowledgment of the overflow that nature gives. The avocado, with its supplement thick profile, turns into a wellspring of appreciation, an affirmation of the healthy food it offers.

The excursion into avocado insight reaches out to the specialty of careful choice. Picking avocados at the pinnacle of readiness includes a material commitment — a delicate press to survey solidness and a nuanced perception of variety changes. In this careful demonstration, people associate with the existence pattern of the natural product, appreciating the persistence expected for ideal maturing.

The act of careful eating inside the setting of avocado insight includes a purposeful interruption before the principal chomp. At this time of tranquility, people develop a familiarity with the tangible components that go with the demonstration of eating. The smooth surface of the avocado, the natural fragrance, and the unpretentious exchange of flavors become an ensemble of vibes that anchor the brain to the current second.

Avocado insight likewise embraces the idea of "eating the rainbow." Past the monochromatic green of avocados, the training empowers a different and beautiful exhibit of leafy foods on the plate. This festival of dietary variety lines up with the standards of care, as each tone addresses an extraordinary arrangement of phytonutrients and medical advantages.

The healthful profile of avocados adjusts agreeably with the standards of a fair and supporting eating routine. Wealthy in heart-solid monounsaturated fats, avocados add to satiety and backing the assimilation of fat-dissolvable nutrients. They additionally give a variety of fundamental supplements, including potassium, nutrients K, C, E, and B-complex nutrients. The fiber content of avocados upholds stomach related wellbeing and manages glucose levels.

With regards to avocado insight, the idea of "appreciation for overflow" turns into a core value. The avocado, with its smooth surface and adaptable culinary applications, represents the overflow of nature's contributions. Offering thanks for the sustenance got from avocados stretches out past the nourishing domain to envelop the social, natural, and social components of food.

Avocado insight urges people to investigate the social meaning of avocados in various foods. From guacamole in Mexican food to avocado toast in contemporary breakfast drifts, the natural product rises above social limits, turning into a flexible and celebrated fixing. This investigation encourages a feeling of social appreciation and an acknowledgment of the different culinary practices that consolidate avocados.

In the embroidery of avocado insight, the biological impression of food decisions arises as a point of convergence. Careful eating includes a consciousness of the natural effect related with food creation and transportation. Avocado insight stretches out past the singular plate to envelop economical and moral works on, provoking people to think about the beginnings of their food and the more extensive ramifications of their dietary decisions.

The excursion into avocado insight welcomes people to investigate the idea of "careful cooking." The readiness of dinners including avocados turns into a purposeful demonstration — an innovative articulation of culinary masterfulness. From making avocado servings of mixed greens to mixing smoothies, the interaction includes drawing in with the energetic varieties, surfaces, and kinds of the natural product with careful consideration.

Avocado insight additionally stretches out its impact to the mutual and social elements of sustenance. Sharing a dinner that highlights avocados turns into a token of association, a method for praising the lavishness of food and cultivate securities inside networks. The demonstration of fellowshipping together, with avocados at the middle, rises above the value-based nature of eating and turns into a common encounter of overflow.

In the investigation of avocado insight, the idea of "careful guilty pleasure" unfurls as a nuanced way to deal with treats and liberal food varieties. Avocado-based pastries, for example, chocolate avocado mousse, become a sweet extravagance as well as a festival of the healthy wealth that avocados offer. Careful extravagance includes relishing these treats with mindfulness and goal, developing a virtuous satisfaction in extraordinary delights.

The blend of avocado insight with the standards of instinctive eating turns into a unique investigation of the body's normal signs and rhythms. Instinctive eating includes adjusting to craving and completion signals, confiding in the body's insight, and developing a positive relationship with food. Avocado insight adjusts consistently with these standards, empowering people to pay attention to their bodies and pursue sustaining decisions in light of interior prompts.

In the domain of careful sustenance, the act of "eating with expectation" turns into a core value. This purposeful methodology includes adjusting one's dietary decisions to individual qualities, wellbeing objectives, and moral contemplations. Avocado insight urges people to move toward their dietary choices with goal, perceiving the interconnectedness between private prosperity and the more extensive setting of food decisions.

The embroidered artwork of avocado insight unfurls further as people investigate the idea of "careful variation." This versatile methodology includes perceiving that wholesome necessities differ in view of variables, for example, age, movement levels, and ailments. Avocado insight welcomes people to develop an adaptable and responsive relationship with their bodies, changing wholesome decisions in light of the powerful idea of prosperity.

As people navigate the scene of avocado insight, the idea of "careful reflection" turns into an extraordinary practice. This intelligent investigation includes occasionally stopping to survey one's relationship with food, recognizing designs, and recognizing the developing idea of nourishing necessities. Careful reflection turns into a compass that guides people towards a more profound comprehension of the multifaceted transaction between psyche, body, and sustenance.

In the coordination of avocado insight into the texture of day to day existence, the act of "careful quietness" arises as a pensive investigation of the physiological cycles engaged with separating and absorbing supplements. In a culture where feasts are in many cases joined by outside improvements, for example, TV or electronic gadgets, the act of careful quietness includes enjoying each nibble with centered consideration. This purposeful quietness makes a safe-haven for the faculties, permitting people to draw in with the tactile experience of eating completely.

The excursion of interfacing care and nourishment through avocado insight reaches out past the person to include cultural and ecological aspects. Careful eating turns into an impetus for cognizant customer decisions, rousing people to help moral and supportable food rehearses. This gradually expanding influence stretches out past private prosperity to add to the aggregate prosperity of the planet.

In the consistently developing scene of careful nourishment, the idea of "careful flexibility" arises as a strengthening force. This strong methodology includes recognizing that the excursion towards comprehensive wellbeing might experience difficulties, mishaps, and variances. Avocado insight, as a foundation of careful flexibility, welcomes people to develop a merciful relationship with themselves, perceiving that prosperity is a dynamic and advancing cycle.

All in all, developing a solid relationship with food through avocado insight divulges an embroidery of interconnectedness — an energetic transaction between psyche, body, and sustenance. The excursion towards all encompassing wellbeing includes the utilization of supplements as well as a careful consciousness of the whole eating experience. Through practices like careful eating, appreciation, and supportable sustenance, people set out on a groundbreaking investigation that rises above the bounds of regular dietary ideal models. In this rich embroidery, each nibble turns into a snapshot of sustenance, a festival of overflow, and a stage towards a more careful and satisfying life.

6

Chapter 5

Avocado in Traditional Medicine

Avocado, experimentally known as Persea Yankee folklore, is a flexible natural product that has acquired huge prominence in contemporary food for its smooth surface and particular flavor. Be that as it may, its importance reaches out past the domain of culinary enjoyments, as the avocado has a rich history well established in conventional medication.

Across different societies and developments, the avocado has been respected for its wellbeing advancing properties. In conventional Mexican medication, avocados were utilized to treat a horde of sicknesses, going from stomach related issues to skin conditions. The organic product's restorative potential was tackled by native networks who perceived its worth in keeping up with generally speaking prosperity.

One of the key components that render avocados valuable in conventional medication is their dietary structure. Plentiful in fundamental supplements like nutrients, minerals, and solid fats, avocados offer an all encompassing way to deal with wellbeing. The presence of monounsaturated fats, explicitly oleic corrosive, adds to the organic product's heart-sound credits, supporting cardiovascular prosperity.

Past the cardiovascular framework, avocados have been customarily utilized to address stomach related concerns. The organic product's high fiber content advances stomach related consistency and forestalls obstruction. Customary healers perceived the significance of a solid stomach related framework in keeping up with generally speaking wellbeing and used avocados as a characteristic solution for address gastrointestinal issues.

Notwithstanding its part in assimilation, avocados were generally used for their calming properties. The presence of mixtures like polyphenols and flavonoids adds to the natural product's capacity to decrease irritation, giving alleviation to conditions portrayed by unnecessary aggravation. This calming impact was outfit in customary medication to mitigate side effects related with joint pain and other fiery problems.

The avocado's effect on skin wellbeing has likewise been a point of convergence in customary restorative practices. The organic product's rich substance of nutrients E and C, alongside monounsaturated fats, adds to its saturating and sustaining properties. Native societies perceived these characteristics and integrated avocados into effective applications, utilizing them to alleviate and hydrate the skin.

Besides, avocados have been generally connected with upgrading fruitfulness and conceptive wellbeing. In certain societies, the organic product was viewed as a love potion, accepted to help drive and work on conceptive capability. Conventional healers frequently suggested avocados as a component of dietary mediations for couples looking to improve their possibilities of origination.

The avocado's part in customary medication isn't restricted to its natural product alone. Different pieces of the avocado tree, including the leaves and seeds, have been used for their restorative properties. Implantations produced using avocado leaves were utilized to resolve issues, for example, hypertension and diabetes. The seeds, wealthy in cancer prevention agents, were utilized for their capability to help safe capability and battle oxidative pressure.

As customary restorative practices have advanced over the long run, mainstream researchers has started to investigate and approve the remedial properties credited to avocados. Present day research has affirmed a considerable lot of the customary purposes of avocados and revealed insight into the components fundamental their wellbeing advancing impacts.

Studies have demonstrated the way that the monounsaturated fats in avocados can decidedly affect cholesterol levels, decreasing the gamble of cardiovascular sicknesses. The natural product's high fiber content has been connected to worked on stomach related wellbeing, with likely advantages for conditions like bad tempered gut disorder (IBS) and diverticulitis.

The calming properties of avocados have additionally been validated by logical examination. Intensifies like polyphenols and carotenoids found in avocados add to their mitigating impacts, making them possibly important in the administration of fiery circumstances like rheumatoid joint pain.

In the domain of skin wellbeing, logical examinations have upheld the possibility that avocados can add to skin hydration and flexibility. The nutrients and fats present in avocados assume a part in keeping up with the skin's obstruction capability and safeguarding it from natural stressors.

The richness upgrading properties credited to avocados in conventional medication have ignited interest in logical examination. While additional examinations are expected to lay out an immediate connection between avocado utilization and fruitfulness, the wholesome profile of avocados proposes that they can add to generally regenerative wellbeing.

As the logical comprehension of avocados keeps on growing, so does their joining into current health rehearses. Avocado-based items, going from skincare plans to dietary enhancements, have become progressively predominant in the wellbeing and health market. This developing pattern reflects not just the ubiquity of avocados as a superfood yet additionally the acknowledgment of their customary restorative roots.

It is fundamental to recognize that while avocados offer various medical advantages, their utilization ought to be important for a reasonable and differed diet. Likewise with any food or regular cure, individual reactions might shift, and talking with medical services experts is prudent, particularly for those with existing ailments or concerns.

All in all, the avocado's excursion from customary medication to standard appreciation is a demonstration of its wonderful flexibility and wellbeing advancing properties. As we keep on investigating the convergence of custom and science in the domain of normal cures, the avocado stands as an image of the getting through shrewdness implanted in conventional restorative practices. Embracing the illustrations of the past while propelling our comprehension through present day research permits us to completely see the value in the all encompassing advantages that nature, in the entirety of its extravagance, brings to the table.

5.1 Historical uses of avocados in traditional healing practices

Since forever ago, avocados play had a huge impact in conventional mending rehearses across different societies. The natural product, experimentally known as Persea Yankee folklore, has been regarded for its culinary allure as well as for its helpful properties. As we dive into the verifiable purposes of avocados in customary recuperating, it becomes obvious that their worth reaches out a long ways past the kitchen, enveloping a scope of physical and profound prosperity.

In old Mesoamerican civilizations, where avocados are accepted to have started, the natural product held a unique spot in conventional recuperating. The Aztecs, for example, adored avocados for their apparent Spanish fly properties. It was accepted that the organic product could upgrade charisma and fruitfulness, prompting its relationship with adoration and sentiment in Aztec culture.

Past issues of the heart, avocados were additionally used for their restorative ascribes. In customary Mexican medication, different pieces of the avocado tree, including the leaves, bark, and seeds, were utilized to address a variety of wellbeing concerns. Implantations produced using avocado leaves were controlled to reduce side effects of conditions like looseness of the bowels and diarrhea. The leaves were additionally accepted to have properties that could help with the administration of hypertension.

The utilization of avocado seeds in conventional mending rehearses was normal by the same token. Wealthy in cancer prevention agents, the seeds were ground into powders or concentrates and used for their capability to battle oxidative pressure and backing safe capability. The comprehensive way to deal with mending that consolidated various pieces of the avocado tree mirrors the interconnectedness of nature and its assorted contributions in conventional medication.

Getting across societies, avocados tracked down their direction into the customary recuperating practices of other native networks. In Focal and South America, avocado leaves were utilized to make implantations accepted to have diuretic properties, supporting the end of abundance liquids from the body. Such practices feature the complex uses of avocados in tending to explicit illnesses as well as advancing by and large health.

In West Africa, avocados were generally utilized for their mitigating properties. Customary healers perceived the capability of avocados to lessen irritation, offering alleviation for conditions like joint pain. The joining of avocados into the conventional pharmacopeia of different societies highlights the comprehensiveness of the natural product's allure chasing after wellbeing and prosperity.

Notwithstanding their inward applications, avocados were used remotely for skin health management in customary mending rehearses. The supporting properties of avocados, credited to their substance of nutrients E and C, as well as monounsaturated fats, made them important in tending to different skin conditions. Avocado-based poultices and treatments were applied topically to calm and saturate the skin, mirroring a comprehension of the natural product's true capacity in advancing dermatological wellbeing.

The customary utilization of avocados in otherworldly and stately settings further underlines the natural product's importance past its actual mending properties. In a few native societies, avocados were viewed as consecrated and utilized in customs to summon endowments and security.

The representative significance of avocados in these social practices addresses the otherworldly association among people and the regular world, rising above the limits of ordinary medication.

As European travelers experienced avocados during their journeys to the Americas, the organic product's standing as a significant restorative asset spread past its landmass of beginning. The exchange of information about the purposes of avocados in customary recuperating rehearses added to the organic product's rising acknowledgment on a worldwide scale.

In the domain of customary Chinese medication, which has a rich history going back millennia, avocados were not local to the district. Notwithstanding, as information on the natural product arrived at Chinese professionals, avocados were integrated into home grown definitions. The conventional Chinese medication point of view frequently centers around the adjusting of energies inside the body, and avocados were accepted to have properties that could blend and feed different organ frameworks.

The flexibility of avocados in different social and geological settings highlights their adaptability in customary mending rehearses. Whether utilized for their dietary benefit, mitigating impacts, or profound importance, avocados have flawlessly coordinated into the texture of conventional medication across the ages.

As we change to the cutting edge time, logical investigation has revealed insight into the substance constituents of avocados, giving a premise to figuring out their conventional purposes. Research has affirmed the presence of bioactive mixtures in avocados, including carotenoids, tocopherols, and polyphenols, which add to their wellbeing advancing impacts.

One of the prominent parts of avocados is oleic corrosive, a monounsaturated fat that is likewise bountiful in olive oil. Oleic corrosive has been related with cardiovascular wellbeing, and studies have shown that it might assist with lessening levels of awful cholesterol (LDL) while expanding levels of good cholesterol (HDL). The cardiovascular advantages ascribed to avocados in customary mending rehearses track down help in contemporary logical discoveries.

The calming properties of avocados, a foundation of their conventional use in tending to conditions like joint pain, have been validated by logical exploration. Mixtures, for example, polyphenols and carotenoids add to the organic product's capacity to regulate fiery reactions in the body. This calming activity lines up with current ways to deal with overseeing ongoing provocative circumstances.

Avocados' effect on skin wellbeing, one more perspective featured in conventional mending, has gathered consideration in the area of dermatology. The mix of nutrients E and C, alongside monounsaturated fats, adds to the organic product's capability to feed and safeguard the skin.

Avocado oil, extricated from the organic product, is presently a famous fixing in skincare items, validating the getting through importance of conventional insight in the excellence and wellbeing industry.

The fruitfulness upgrading properties ascribed to avocados in conventional medication have provoked logical request. While more examination is expected to lay out an immediate connection between avocado utilization and fruitfulness, the wholesome profile of avocados recommends likely advantages for regenerative wellbeing. Supplements like folate, vitamin E, and solid fats assume critical parts in supporting by and large fruitfulness, and avocados can add to meeting these nourishing requirements.

The shift from conventional purposes of avocados to their mix into present day wellbeing rehearses has been set apart by the development of avocado-based items and enhancements. Avocado oil, known for its culinary and skincare applications, has turned into a staple in wellbeing cognizant families. Avocado enhancements, embodying the nourishing decency of the organic product, take special care of those looking for helpful ways of integrating avocados into their day to day schedules.

While the investigation of avocados in conventional mending rehearses has prepared for their acknowledgment in standard wellbeing cognizance, moving toward their utilization with a fair perspective is fundamental. Likewise with any normal cure or dietary intercession, individual reactions might change. Talking with medical services experts, particularly for those with existing ailments or concerns, is prudent to guarantee that avocados supplement an individual's general wellbeing and health plan.

All in all, the verifiable purposes of avocados in customary mending rehearses offer a captivating excursion through time, revealing the different manners by which this organic product has been esteemed for its restorative and profound importance. From antiquated civic establishments to the current day, avocados have risen above social limits, meshing themselves into the embroidered artwork of human prosperity. The intermingling of conventional insight and current logical figuring out features the getting through pertinence of avocados as a comprehensive asset for wellbeing, exemplifying the interconnectedness of nature and human prospering.

5.2 Modern scientific perspectives on the medicinal properties of avocados

As of late, established researchers has progressively directed its concentration toward the restorative properties of avocados, looking to approve and figure out the conventional purposes of this flexible natural product. Present day research has given an abundance of data, revealing insight into the biochemical sythesis of avocados and the instruments behind their potential medical advantages.

One of the critical parts of avocados that has accumulated logical interest is their dietary profile. Avocados are wealthy in monounsaturated fats, especially oleic corrosive, which is likewise tracked down in olive oil. These sound fats have been related with cardiovascular advantages. Studies have shown that the monounsaturated fats in avocados might assist with bringing down degrees of low-thickness lipoprotein (LDL) cholesterol, frequently alluded to as "awful" cholesterol, while expanding high-thickness lipoprotein (HDL) cholesterol, the "upside" cholesterol. This lipid profile balance adds to heart wellbeing, lining up with the authentic utilization of avocados in customary medication for cardiovascular help.

Past fats, avocados are a supplement force to be reckoned with, containing a variety of nutrients and minerals. They are especially plentiful in potassium, a fundamental mineral for keeping up with sound pulse levels. The potassium content in avocados, combined with their low sodium content, upholds a positive sodium-potassium balance in the body, which is vital for cardiovascular wellbeing. The logical investigation of these dietary viewpoints gives a strong groundwork to understanding the cardiovascular advantages related with avocado utilization.

Notwithstanding their cardiovascular effect, avocados have been researched for their part in advancing stomach related wellbeing. The high fiber content of avocados adds to their true capacity in supporting customary solid discharges and forestalling blockage. Dietary fiber is known to add mass to the stool, working with its development through the gastrointestinal system. The dissolvable fiber in avocados may likewise add to a sensation of completion, which can be helpful for weight the executives. As present day research dives into the multifaceted connections among avocados and the gastrointestinal framework, it reaffirms the conventional utilization of avocados in tending to stomach related concerns.

The calming properties of avocados, a trademark featured in customary medication, have been a subject of logical examination. Constant irritation is ensnared in different ailments, including cardiovascular sicknesses, joint pain, and certain metabolic problems. Avocados contain bioactive mixtures, for example, polyphenols and carotenoids, which have been displayed to make calming impacts. These mixtures adjust the provocative pathways in the body, possibly offering restorative advantages in the administration of fiery circumstances. The combination of conventional insight and logical proof in such manner highlights the all encompassing capability of avocados in advancing in general prosperity.

Avocados' effect on skin wellbeing, a feature perceived in conventional recuperating rehearses, has tracked down approval in present day dermatological examination. The mix of nutrients E and C, alongside monounsaturated fats, adds to the natural product's saturating and cell reinforcement properties. Avocado oil, extricated from the natural product, is wealthy in these gainful parts and has been integrated into skincare definitions. Studies have demonstrated the way that effective use of avocado oil can upgrade skin hydration, further develop versatility, and shield the skin from natural harm.

This logical comprehension lines up with the verifiable utilization of avocados for effective applications in customary medication, reaffirming the natural product's job in dermatological wellbeing.

The fruitfulness upgrading properties credited to avocados in customary medication have provoked logical investigation into their likely effect on conceptive wellbeing. While research in this space is progressing, the nourishing parts of avocados propose potential advantages for ripeness. Folate, a B-nutrient present in avocados, is pivotal for fetal turn of events and is frequently suggested for ladies during pregnancy. Also, the by and large wholesome lavishness of avocados upholds general conceptive wellbeing. The interdisciplinary methodology of consolidating customary information with present day logical procedures adds to a more thorough comprehension of avocados' expected job in richness.

As scientists dig into the atomic instruments fundamental the wellbeing advancing impacts of avocados, they have recognized the presence of bioactive mixtures with cancer prevention agent properties. Cancer prevention agents assume an imperative part in killing free revolutionaries, which are shaky atoms that can cause cell harm and add to maturing and different sicknesses. The cell reinforcements in avocados, including carotenoids and tocopherols, add to the natural product's capacity to battle oxidative pressure. This antioxidative limit lines up with the conventional utilization of avocados in customary mending rehearses, where they were utilized for their capability to balance the impacts of ecological stressors on the body.

The investigation of avocados with regards to metabolic wellbeing has additionally yielded intriguing discoveries. Avocados might play a part in glucose guideline, making them possibly useful for people with diabetes or those in danger of fostering the condition. The monounsaturated fats and solvent fiber in avocados add to their capacity to tweak blood glucose levels. Studies have shown that integrating avocados into dinners can prompt better post-feast glucose reactions. This part of avocado examination lines up with the more extensive comprehension of the organic product's effect on metabolic wellbeing, consolidating customary experiences with contemporary logical procedures.

The bioavailability of supplements from avocados has been one more area of logical interest. A few supplements, like fat-dissolvable nutrients (e.g., vitamin E), are better caught up within the sight of dietary fats. The sound fats in avocados might upgrade the assimilation of these fat-dissolvable nutrients, adding to the general supplement thickness of the organic product. This nuanced comprehension of supplement retention adds a layer of intricacy to the customary information on avocados as a healthfully thick food.

The worldwide interest in avocados has provoked specialists to investigate various assortments of the organic product, each with its remarkable structure. For instance, Hass avocados, quite possibly of the most well known assortment, have been widely read up for their nourishing

substance and potential medical advantages. Understanding the varieties in supplement profiles among various avocado assortments considers more designated suggestions in light of individual wellbeing objectives.

In the domain of disease research, avocados stand out enough to be noticed for their potential enemy of malignant growth properties. A few examinations recommend that specific mixtures in avocados might have a defensive impact against malignant growth cells. The cell reinforcement and calming properties of avocados, combined with their commitment to generally cell wellbeing, add to their true capacity in disease counteraction. While more examination is expected to lay out authoritative ends, the starter discoveries line up with the all encompassing way to deal with wellbeing pushed in customary recuperating rehearses.

As current logical points of view on the restorative properties of avocados keep on developing, perceiving the interdisciplinary idea of this exploration is essential. The intermingling of dietary science, natural chemistry, dermatology, and different fields adds to a far reaching comprehension of what avocados mean for human wellbeing. This cooperative methodology takes into consideration a nuanced translation of the customary purposes of avocados, incorporating old insight with contemporary logical systems.

The interpretation of logical discoveries into functional proposals has prompted the consideration of avocados in dietary rules for advancing heart wellbeing, overseeing weight, and supporting in general prosperity. The adaptability of avocados in culinary applications, from servings of mixed greens to smoothies, makes it helpful for people to integrate this supplement thick organic product into their everyday eating regimens.

In any case, it means a lot to move toward the utilization of avocados, similar to any food or supplement, with a fair viewpoint. While they offer various medical advantages, individual reactions might shift. The setting of one's general dietary example, way of life, and wellbeing status ought to be thought of. Talking with medical care experts, particularly for those with explicit wellbeing concerns or conditions, guarantees that the consolidation of avocados lines up with customized wellbeing objectives.

Avocados, experimentally known as Persea Yankee folklore, have risen above their customary culinary job to arise as a subject of broad examination inferable from their likely restorative properties. This flexible organic product, local to Focal and South America, has a rich history profoundly entwined with conventional recuperating rehearses. As we dive into the restorative properties of avocados, it becomes obvious that their wholesome extravagance and bioactive mixtures certainly stand out across different logical disciplines.

A foundation of the restorative worth credited to avocados lies in their extraordinary nourishing sythesis. Avocados are prestigious for their high satisfied of monounsaturated fats, dominatingly oleic corrosive.

This kind of sound fat, likewise found in olive oil, has been related with cardiovascular advantages. Research shows that the utilization of monounsaturated fats might add to a positive lipid profile by lessening levels of low-thickness lipoprotein (LDL) cholesterol, ordinarily alluded to as "terrible" cholesterol, while expanding high-thickness lipoprotein (HDL) cholesterol, known as "great" cholesterol. These lipid-regulating properties line up with the authentic utilization of avocados in customary medication for supporting heart wellbeing.

Notwithstanding solid fats, avocados brag a noteworthy exhibit of nutrients and minerals. Potassium, an imperative mineral for keeping up with circulatory strain levels, is plentiful in avocados. The harmony among potassium and sodium is pivotal for cardiovascular wellbeing, and avocados' potassium-rich profile adds to this balance. The logical investigation of avocados' wholesome substance gives a vigorous establishment to figuring out their possible effect on cardiovascular prosperity, lining up with conventional practices that perceived the natural product's importance in heart wellbeing.

The job of avocados in advancing stomach related wellbeing has likewise turned into a point of convergence of logical request. The high fiber content in avocados adds to their true capacity in supporting ordinary defecations and forestalling blockage. Dietary fiber, fundamental for stomach related routineness, adds mass to the stool and works with its entry through the gastrointestinal parcel. This part of avocado exploration reverberates with conventional purposes, where avocados were generally utilized to address gastrointestinal worries. The cooperative energy between customary information and present day logical approval underscores the comprehensive advantages avocados proposition to the stomach related framework.

The calming properties of avocados, a trademark featured in conventional mending rehearses, have been a subject of sharp logical interest. Ongoing aggravation is ensnared in different ailments, including cardiovascular sicknesses, joint pain, and metabolic problems. Avocados contain bioactive mixtures, for example, polyphenols and carotenoids, which make showed calming impacts. These mixtures balance fiery pathways, introducing expected helpful advantages in overseeing provocative circumstances. The agreeable coordination of customary thinking and logical proof highlights avocados' all encompassing potential in advancing by and large prosperity.

Avocados' positive effect on skin wellbeing, a feature perceived in customary medicine, has tracked down validation in present day dermatological examination. The mix of nutrients E and C, alongside monounsaturated fats, adds to the organic product's saturating and cell reinforcement properties. Avocado oil, got from the natural product, has turned into a famous fixing in skincare details. Logical investigations affirm that effective use of avocado oil upgrades skin hydration, further develops versatility, and safeguards the skin from natural harm. This logical approval lines up with authentic practices that used avocados for their dermatological advantages, featuring the organic product's part in skin wellbeing.

The fruitfulness upgrading properties credited to avocados in customary medication have provoked logical investigation into their possible effect on conceptive wellbeing. While progressing research means to lay out an immediate connection between avocado utilization and ripeness, the nourishing parts of avocados recommend likely advantages for regenerative wellbeing. Folate, a B-nutrient present in avocados, is pivotal for fetal turn of events and is suggested for ladies during pregnancy. The thorough methodology of consolidating conventional information with present day logical philosophies adds to a nuanced comprehension of avocados' possible job in richness.

The cell reinforcement properties of avocados, significant for battling oxidative pressure, have been a point of convergence in logical examinations. Cell reinforcements assume a vital part in killing free extremists, unsteady particles that can cause cell harm and add to maturing and different sicknesses. Avocados contain cell reinforcements like carotenoids and tocopherols, adding to their capacity to neutralize oxidative pressure. This lines up with the customary utilization of avocados in conventional recuperating rehearses, where they were utilized for their capability to alleviate the impacts of natural stressors on the body.

With regards to metabolic wellbeing, avocados possibly affect glucose guideline. The monounsaturated fats and solvent fiber in avocados add to their capacity to balance blood glucose levels. Research shows that integrating avocados into dinners can prompt better post-feast glucose reactions. This aspect of avocado exploration lines up with the more extensive comprehension of the natural product's effect on metabolic wellbeing, incorporating customary experiences with contemporary logical systems.

The bioavailability of supplements from avocados has additionally aroused logical curiosity. Certain supplements, particularly fat-dissolvable nutrients like vitamin E, are better caught up within the sight of dietary fats. The solid fats in avocados might upgrade the retention of these nutrients, adding to the general supplement thickness of the organic product. This nuanced comprehension of supplement retention adds profundity to conventional information, recognizing avocados as a healthfully thick food.

Various assortments of avocados have been considered to figure out varieties in supplement profiles. For instance, the Hass avocado, a well known assortment, has been broadly broke down for its dietary substance and potential medical advantages. Perceiving these varieties takes into consideration more designated suggestions in view of individual wellbeing objectives.

In the domain of disease research, avocados stand out for their potential enemy of malignant growth properties. A few examinations recommend that specific mixtures in avocados might have a defensive impact against malignant growth cells. The cancer prevention agent and calming properties of avocados, combined with their commitment to generally cell wellbeing, add to their true capacity in disease counteraction.

While more exploration is expected to lay out authoritative ends, the starter discoveries line up with the all encompassing way to deal with wellbeing supported in customary mending rehearses.

As present day logical points of view on the restorative properties of avocados keep on advancing, perceiving the interdisciplinary idea of this exploration is significant. The combination of dietary science, organic chemistry, dermatology, and different fields adds to a complete comprehension of what avocados mean for human wellbeing. This cooperative methodology takes into consideration a nuanced translation of the customary purposes of avocados, coordinating old insight with contemporary logical procedures.

The interpretation of logical discoveries into down to earth proposals has prompted the consideration of avocados in dietary rules for advancing heart wellbeing, overseeing weight, and supporting in general prosperity. The adaptability of avocados in culinary applications, from plates of mixed greens to smoothies, makes it advantageous for people to integrate this supplement thick natural product into their day to day consumes less calories.

Nonetheless, it means quite a bit to move toward the utilization of avocados, similar to any food or supplement, with a decent point of view. While they offer various medical advantages, individual reactions might change. The setting of one's general dietary example, way of life, and wellbeing status ought to be thought of. Talking with medical services experts, particularly for those with explicit wellbeing concerns or conditions, guarantees that the joining of avocados lines up with customized wellbeing objectives.

5.3 Integrating avocado wisdom into holistic well-being

The reconciliation of avocado insight into all encompassing prosperity incorporates a complete methodology that recognizes the verifiable, conventional, and present day components of this flexible natural product's effect on human wellbeing. Avocados, logically known as Persea History of the U.S, have crossed through hundreds of years of conventional recuperating rehearses and culinary applications to arise as an image of comprehensive health. In investigating the coordination of avocado insight into all encompassing prosperity, we explore through the domains of nourishment, conventional medication, current science, and careful living.

At the core of this reconciliation is a comprehension of the nourishing lavishness that avocados offer. Past their culinary allure, avocados are supplement forces to be reckoned with, giving a variety of nutrients, minerals, and solid fats. The monounsaturated fats, especially oleic corrosive, add to heart wellbeing by tweaking cholesterol levels. The high potassium content backings cardiovascular prosperity by keeping up with solid circulatory strain levels. The nutrients E and C, alongside cancer prevention agents like carotenoids, add to skin wellbeing and battle oxidative pressure. Embracing avocado insight includes perceiving and integrating these wholesome advantages into a comprehensive way to deal with prosperity.

Conventional recuperating rehearses have long loved avocados for their different helpful properties. From addressing stomach related worries to advancing skin wellbeing and richness, avocados have been woven into the texture of customary medication across societies. The utilization of various pieces of the avocado tree, including leaves, bark, and seeds, in customary cures mirrors an all encompassing comprehension of the interconnectedness among nature and human wellbeing. The coordination of avocado insight into comprehensive prosperity requires embracing the customary information that has endured everyday hardship.

Present day logical points of view on avocados have approved numerous customary purposes while revealing new components of their wellbeing advancing impacts. Research has validated the cardiovascular advantages of avocados, affirming their part in lipid profile adjustment and circulatory strain guideline. The mitigating and cell reinforcement properties of avocados, featured in customary recuperating, have tracked down help in logical examinations, giving a premise to figuring out their true capacity in overseeing fiery circumstances and fighting oxidative pressure. The joining of avocado insight into comprehensive prosperity requires an appreciation for the marriage of old experiences with contemporary logical approval.

In the domain of skincare, the reconciliation of avocado insight includes perceiving the organic product's part in advancing dermatological wellbeing. Avocado oil, plentiful in nutrients and monounsaturated fats, has turned into a sought-after fixing in skincare definitions. Logical investigations assert the saturating, sustaining, and defensive properties of avocado oil on the skin. The customary utilization of avocados for effective applications lines up with present day skincare works on, stressing the comprehensive way to deal with keeping up with solid and brilliant skin.

The ripeness upgrading properties credited to avocados in customary medication brief a nuanced investigation of their part in conceptive wellbeing. While research is continuous to lay out an immediate connection between avocado utilization and richness, the dietary parts of avocados propose expected benefits for regenerative prosperity. Incorporating avocado insight into comprehensive prosperity includes considering the wholesome help that avocados can accommodate generally speaking regenerative wellbeing, perceiving their commitment to a decent and supplement rich eating regimen.

Careful living is a urgent part of incorporating avocado insight into comprehensive prosperity. Avocados, with their energetic green shade and supporting properties, welcome an association with nature and a cognizant way to deal with sustaining the body and brain. Careful eating, which includes enjoying each chomp and being available at the time, lines up with the soul of all encompassing prosperity. Picking avocados as a feature of a fair and fluctuated diet turns into a careful choice, appreciating their taste as well as their likely commitments to by and large wellbeing.

The flexibility of avocados in culinary applications improves their reconciliation into comprehensive prosperity. From flavorful dishes to smoothies and treats, avocados loan themselves to a heap of arrangements that take care of different preferences and inclinations. The mix of avocado insight into comprehensive prosperity includes investigating innovative and nutritious ways of integrating avocados into feasts, advancing both actual sustenance and culinary happiness.

With regards to comprehensive prosperity, recognizing individual varieties and the significance of customized approaches is fundamental. Avocado utilization might communicate diversely with different medical issue or dietary inclinations. Talking with medical care experts guarantees that the coordination of avocado insight lines up with a singular's one of a kind wellbeing objectives and prerequisites.

Ecological awareness is a necessary piece of comprehensive prosperity, and avocados deliver contemplations connected with maintainability. The developing interest for avocados has raised ecological worries, especially with respect to water utilization in avocado-creating locales. Incorporating avocado insight into all encompassing prosperity includes pursuing informed decisions, supporting maintainable practices, and taking into account the more extensive effect of dietary decisions on the climate.

The reconciliation of avocado insight into comprehensive prosperity stretches out past individual wellbeing to envelop local area prosperity. Avocado-creating districts frequently assume an essential part in neighborhood economies, giving occupations to networks. Supporting maintainable and moral practices in avocado creation adds to the all encompassing prosperity of these networks. Careful utilization includes perceiving the more extensive ramifications of our decisions and pursuing choices that line up with standards of social obligation and moral obtaining.

Comprehensive prosperity additionally envelops mental and profound wellbeing. The tactile experience of getting a charge out of avocados, from their velvety surface to their rich flavor, adds an element of joy to eating. The demonstration of planning and sharing avocado-based feasts can turn into a careful and pleasant custom, encouraging positive feelings and associations. The combination of avocado insight into all encompassing prosperity includes perceiving the potential for food to sustain the body as well as add to mental and close to home prosperity.

The idea of comprehensive prosperity recognizes the interconnectedness of various parts of life, embracing physical, mental, profound, and ecological aspects. Avocado insight, drawn from customary practices and approved by present day science, lines up with this all encompassing methodology. Whether in the kitchen, skincare schedule, or dietary decisions, avocados act as an image of the agreeable reconciliation of old insight and contemporary figuring out chasing all encompassing prosperity.

7

Chapter 6

Growing Your Own Avocado Tree

Developing your own avocado tree can be a fulfilling and fulfilling experience, permitting you to partake in the your rewards for all the hard work, straightforwardly. Avocado trees, logically known as Persea Yankee folklore, are local to Focal and South America however have become famous in many regions of the planet because of the scrumptious and nutritious organic product they produce.

To leave on the excursion of developing your own avocado tree, you'll require some persistence, devotion, and a fundamental comprehension of the tree's necessities. Avocado trees are tropical and subtropical plants, flourishing in warm environments. Notwithstanding, with the right consideration, they can likewise be filled in pots and compartments, making them reasonable for a more extensive scope of conditions.

The most vital phase in developing your avocado tree is to choose a solid avocado pit from an experienced natural product. Pick a ready avocado, and cautiously eliminate the pit. The pit is the enormous seed in the focal point of the organic product. Flush the pit under running water to eliminate any excess tissue, and wipe it off with a paper towel.

When you have a perfect avocado pit, you'll have to set it up for germination. Many individuals suggest suspending the pit over a glass of water utilizing toothpicks. Embed three or four toothpicks around the center of the pit, equally dispersed, and afterward put the toothpicks on the edge of the glass, permitting the lower part of the pit to be lowered in water.

Change the water routinely, and inside half a month, you ought to begin to see roots rising up out of the lower part of the pit. This denotes the start of the germination cycle. It's critical to take note of that not all avocado pits will effectively develop, so it's really smart to begin with different pits to build your odds of coming out on top.

When the roots are a couple inches long, you can move the sprouted pit to a pot with soil. Utilize a well-depleting preparing blend, and plant the pit with the sharp end looking vertical. Keep the dirt reliably damp yet not waterlogged, as avocados don't endure spongy circumstances.

As your avocado seedling develops, it will foster leaves, and you can step by step adapt it to more daylight. Avocado trees flourish in full sun, so giving them satisfactory light is fundamental for their general wellbeing and efficiency. On the off chance that you're developing your avocado tree inside, setting it close to a south-bound window can assist with guaranteeing it gets adequate daylight.

Appropriate watering is critical being taken care of by avocado trees. While they favor reliably damp soil, overwatering can prompt root decay, a typical issue that can undermine the wellbeing of your tree. Then again, permitting the dirt to dry out totally can pressure the plant. Finding the right equilibrium is vital to fruitful avocado tree care.

Preparing your avocado tree is likewise significant, particularly on the off chance that it's filling in a holder. Pick a reasonable manure with equivalent measures of nitrogen, phosphorus, and potassium. Apply the compost as indicated by the maker's guidelines, and screen the tree's reaction. Over-preparing can prompt salt development in the dirt, unfavorably influencing the tree.

Pruning is one more part of avocado tree care that can add to its general wellbeing and shape. Standard pruning keeps a reasonable size, supports stretching, and eliminates dead or harmed development. Be that as it may, unreasonable pruning ought to be kept away from, as it can pressure the tree.

As your avocado tree develops, it will probably begin creating blossoms. Avocado trees are novel in that they have both male and female blossoms on a similar tree, however they regularly don't self-fertilize. To guarantee organic product creation, you might require various avocado trees or support the presence of pollinators like honey bees.

The time it takes for an avocado tree to prove to be fruitful can fluctuate. A few trees might begin delivering natural product inside a couple of years, while others might take more time. Factors like the tree's age, wellbeing, and developing circumstances all assume a part in organic product improvement.

Persistence is key while developing avocados, as it can require quite a long while for a tree to arrive at development and produce critical organic product yields. Nonetheless, the stand by is much of the time definitely justified, taking into account the fulfillment of collecting your own avocados.

Notwithstanding their tasty taste, avocados are loaded with supplements and medical advantages. They are wealthy in monounsaturated fats, which are heart-sound fats that can assist with bringing down awful cholesterol levels. Avocados likewise give a decent wellspring of nutrients and minerals, including vitamin K, vitamin E, L-ascorbic acid, and different B nutrients.

The adaptability of avocados stretches out past just cutting them for servings of mixed greens or spreading them on toast. They can be utilized in various dishes, from guacamole to smoothies, adding a velvety surface and a wholesome lift. Developing your own avocados permits you to have a new and practical stockpile of this nutritious organic product right readily available.

While the method involved with growing an avocado tree might appear to be direct, it's fundamental to know about possible difficulties and mishaps. Bugs and illnesses can influence avocado trees, so routinely examining your tree for difficult situations is essential. Normal nuisances incorporate aphids, bugs, and scale bugs, while illnesses like root decay and anthracnose can present dangers to the tree's wellbeing.

Carrying out regular and natural irritation control strategies is prudent to limit the utilization of hurtful synthetic substances. Neem oil, insecticidal cleanser, and presenting valuable bugs are successful ways of overseeing nuisances without compromising the wellbeing of your avocado tree.

Notwithstanding bugs and illnesses, natural factors, for example, outrageous temperatures can influence avocado trees. While they flourish in warm environments, they might be powerless to ice and cold temperatures. Assuming you live in a space with periodic cool fronts, safeguarding your avocado tree with ice material or bringing it inside during outrageous weather conditions can assist with guaranteeing its endurance.

Holder developed avocado trees offer the upside of portability, permitting you to move the tree inside during cold seasons and outside during hotter months. This adaptability is especially useful for those living in areas with flighty environments.

To upgrade the progress of your avocado tree, consider sidekick planting. A few plants, like basil and marigolds, are known to repulse bothers that can influence avocado trees. Intercropping these friend plants around your avocado tree can make a stronger and adjusted biological system.

As your avocado tree develops and starts to prove to be fruitful, appropriate reaping is critical to guarantee ideal flavor and quality. Avocados are normally collected when they have arrived at the ideal size and immovability, however they are still marginally green. Ready avocados respect delicate strain when crushed however are not excessively delicate.

Reaping should be possible the hard way, utilizing pruning shears or by curving the natural product tenderly until it withdraws from the stem. It's significant not to pull or tear the natural product from the tree, as this can cause harm and influence future fruiting.

Once reaped, avocados keep on aging off the tree. If you have any desire to defer the maturing system, store the avocados in the fridge. Then again, if you need to accelerate maturing, place the avocados in a paper sack with a banana or apple, as these organic products discharge ethylene gas, a characteristic aging specialist.

As well as appreciating avocados for their culinary allure, you can investigate innovative ways of integrating them into your regular routine. Avocado oil, separated from the natural product, is a nutritious cooking oil with a high smoke point, making it reasonable for different cooking strategies. It likewise tastes gentle that supplements both sweet and appetizing dishes.

Moreover, avocados can be utilized in natively constructed excellence medicines. The normal oils in avocados are great for saturating and feeding the skin and hair. You can make Do-It-Yourself facial coverings, hair veils, and scours utilizing crushed avocado blended in with other regular fixings like honey, yogurt, or oats.

Developing your own avocado tree not just gives you a manageable wellspring of new and nutritious organic product yet in addition associates you to the regular world and the pattern of development. The method involved with sustaining a small seed into a flourishing tree is a strong and satisfying experience that encourages a more profound appreciation for the climate and the food we devour.

All in all, developing your own avocado tree is a compensating try that consolidates cultivation, supportability, and culinary happiness. From choosing a sound pit to really focusing on a full grown tree, each move toward the cycle adds to the general progress of your avocado-developing excursion.

While difficulties might emerge, the fulfillment of reaping local avocados and integrating them into your way of life puts forth the attempt beneficial. Thus, focus in, get some dirt, and begin developing your own avocado tree - a green and heavenly expansion to your home and nursery.

6.1 A guide to cultivating avocados at home

Developing avocados at home can be a satisfying and remunerating experience, offering an immediate association with the wellspring of this famous and nutritious organic product. Avocado trees (Persea Yankee folklore) are local to Focal and South America, however their flexibility has made them a number one among home grounds-keepers all over the planet. Developing avocados at home requires persistence, scrupulousness, and a readiness to find out about the particular necessities of these tropical and subtropical trees.

To begin the interaction, pick a full grown and solid avocado for its pit. The pit is the huge seed found at the focal point of the natural product. Whenever you've chosen a ready avocado, cautiously eliminate the pit and clean it completely under running water. Utilize a paper towel to wipe it off, it is taken out to guarantee all excess tissue. This cleaned pit is the establishment for developing your avocado tree.

The subsequent stage is to set up the avocado pit for germination. Numerous nursery workers select to suspend the pit over a glass of water utilizing toothpicks. Embed three or four toothpicks equitably around the center of the pit and put them on the edge of the glass, permitting the lower part of the pit to submerge in water. Change the water consistently, and following half a month, you ought to notice roots rising up out of the lower part of the pit, flagging the beginning of germination. It's essential to take note of that not all avocado pits will effectively sprout, so it's prudent to begin with a few to improve the probability of progress.

When the roots are a couple inches long, move the developed pit to a pot with well-depleting soil. Utilize a quality preparing blend, and plant the pit with the sharp end looking vertical. Keep up with steady dampness in the dirt without permitting it to become waterlogged, as avocados don't flourish in excessively saturated conditions.

As your avocado seedling develops, it will foster leaves, and you can step by step adapt it to more daylight. Avocado trees flourish in full sun, so furnishing them with sufficient light is vital for their general well-being and efficiency. In the event that you're developing your avocado tree inside, putting it close to a south-bound window can assist with guaranteeing it gets adequate daylight.

Legitimate watering is fundamental being taken care of by avocado trees. While they favor reliably wet soil, overwatering can prompt root decay, a typical issue that can undermine the wellbeing of your tree. Then again, permitting the dirt to dry out totally can pressure the plant. Finding some kind of harmony is critical to effective avocado tree care.

Treating your avocado tree is likewise imperative, particularly in the event that it's filled in a holder. Settle on a reasonable compost with equivalent measures of nitrogen, phosphorus, and potassium. Apply the manure adhering to the producer's directions and screen the tree's reaction. Over-treating can bring about salt development in the dirt, antagonistically influencing the tree.

Pruning assumes a part in avocado tree care by keeping a reasonable size, empowering stretching, and eliminating dead or harmed development. In any case, exorbitant pruning ought to be stayed away from, as it can pressure the tree. Consistently review your tree for indications of nuisances and infections, which can influence its wellbeing. Aphids, parasites, and scale bugs are normal nuisances, while illnesses like root decay and anthracnose present dangers to the tree.

Executing normal and natural bug control strategies is prudent to limit the utilization of hurtful synthetic compounds. Neem oil, insecticidal cleanser, and presenting gainful bugs are compelling ways of overseeing irritations without compromising the strength of your avocado tree.

Natural variables, like outrageous temperatures, can likewise influence avocado trees. While they flourish in warm environments, they might be vulnerable to ice and cold temperatures. Assuming you live in a space with periodic cool spells, safeguarding your avocado tree with ice material or bringing it inside during outrageous weather conditions can assist with guaranteeing its endurance.

Holder developed avocado trees offer the benefit of versatility, permitting you to move the tree inside during cold seasons and outside during hotter months. This adaptability is especially valuable for those living in districts with unusual environments.

Buddy planting can upgrade the outcome of your avocado tree. A few plants, like basil and marigolds, are known to repulse bothers that can influence avocado trees. Intercropping these sidekick plants around your avocado tree can make a stronger and adjusted biological system.

As your avocado tree develops and begins creating blossoms, you might see a special component: avocado trees have both male and female blossoms on a similar tree, yet they normally don't self-fertilize. To guarantee natural product creation, you might require various avocado trees or support the presence of pollinators like honey bees.

The time it takes for an avocado tree to prove to be fruitful can change. A few trees might begin creating natural product inside a couple of years, while others might take more time. Factors like the tree's age, wellbeing, and developing circumstances all assume a part in organic product improvement.

Persistence is a prudence while developing avocados, as it can require quite a long while for a tree to arrive at development and produce critical natural product yields. In any case, the stand by is much of the time definitely justified, taking into account the fulfillment of reaping your own avocados.

Notwithstanding their scrumptious taste, avocados are loaded with supplements and medical advantages. They are wealthy in monounsaturated fats, which are heart-sound fats that can assist with bringing down terrible cholesterol levels. Avocados likewise give a decent wellspring of nutrients and minerals, including vitamin K, vitamin E, L-ascorbic acid, and different B nutrients.

The flexibility of avocados reaches out past basically cutting them for plates of mixed greens or spreading them on toast. They can be utilized in different dishes, from guacamole to smoothies, adding a velvety surface and a healthful lift. Developing your own avocados permits you to have a new and maintainable stock of this nutritious organic product right readily available.

While the method involved with growing an avocado tree might appear to be clear, it's fundamental to know about expected difficulties and mishaps. Irritations and infections can influence avocado trees, so routinely examining your tree for difficult situations is critical. Normal bugs incorporate aphids, vermin, and scale bugs, while infections like root decay and anthracnose can present dangers to the tree's wellbeing.

Executing normal and natural bug control techniques is fitting to limit the utilization of unsafe synthetic compounds. Neem oil, insecticidal cleanser, and presenting valuable bugs are successful ways of overseeing nuisances without compromising the strength of your avocado tree.

Notwithstanding bugs and infections, natural factors, for example, outrageous temperatures can influence avocado trees. While they flourish in warm environments, they might be vulnerable to ice and cold temperatures. Assuming you live in a space with periodic cool spells, safeguarding your avocado tree with ice material or bringing it inside during outrageous weather conditions can assist with guaranteeing its endurance.

Compartment developed avocado trees offer the benefit of portability, permitting you to move the tree inside during cold seasons and outside during hotter months. This adaptability is especially gainful for those living in locales with unusual environments.

To improve the outcome of your avocado tree, consider sidekick planting. A few plants, like basil and marigolds, are known to repulse bothers that can influence avocado trees. Intercropping these friend plants around your avocado tree can make a stronger and adjusted environment.

As your avocado tree develops and starts to prove to be fruitful, legitimate reaping is significant to guarantee ideal flavor and quality. Avocados are normally collected when they have arrived at the ideal size and solidness however are still marginally green. Ready avocados respect delicate strain when pressed however are not excessively delicate.

Collecting should be possible the hard way, utilizing pruning shears or by curving the natural product delicately until it withdraws from the stem. It's significant not to pull or tear the natural product from the tree, as this can cause harm and influence future fruiting.

Once gathered, avocados keep on aging off the tree. If you have any desire to defer the aging system, store the avocados in the cooler. Then again, if you need to accelerate maturing, place the avocados in a paper sack with a banana or apple, as these organic products discharge ethylene gas, a characteristic maturing specialist.

As well as appreciating avocados for their culinary allure, you can investigate innovative ways of integrating them into your regular routine. Avocado oil, extricated from the organic product, is a nutritious cooking oil with a high smoke point, making it reasonable for different cooking techniques. It likewise tastes gentle that supplements both sweet and appetizing dishes.

Moreover, avocados can be utilized in hand crafted excellence medicines. The normal oils in avocados are brilliant for saturating and supporting the skin and hair. You can make Do-It-Yourself facial coverings, hair veils, and cleans utilizing crushed avocado blended in with other regular fixings like honey, yogurt, or cereal.

Developing your own avocado tree not just gives you a manageable wellspring of new and nutritious organic product yet additionally interfaces you to the normal world and the pattern of development. The method involved with supporting a small seed into a flourishing tree is a strong and satisfying experience that encourages a more profound appreciation for the climate and the food we eat.

All in all, developing avocados at home is a remunerating try that consolidates cultivation, maintainability, and culinary happiness. From choosing a solid pit to really focusing on a developed tree, each move toward the cycle adds to the general outcome of your avocado-developing excursion. While difficulties might emerge, the fulfillment of reaping local avocados and integrating them into your way of life puts forth the attempt beneficial. Thus, focus in, snatch some dirt, and begin developing your own avocado tree - a green and delightful expansion to your home and nursery.

6.2 Sustainable practices and environmental benefits

Manageable practices are turning out to be progressively vital in our advanced world as we wrestle with natural difficulties. These practices intend to address the issues of the present without compromising the capacity of people in the future to address their own issues. From farming to energy utilization, feasible practices assume a crucial part in relieving the effect of human exercises on the climate. By embracing and advancing maintainability, we can address environmental change, save biodiversity, and make a better planet for current and people in the future.

One of the key regions where manageable practices are having a tremendous effect is farming. Ordinary horticulture frequently depends on escalated substance inputs, monoculture cultivating, and enormous scope water system, adding to soil corruption, water contamination, and loss of biodiversity. Conversely, supportable farming spotlights on regenerative practices that focus on soil wellbeing, water protection, and biodiversity.

Crop revolution, cover trimming, and agroforestry are instances of supportable rural practices that improve soil fruitfulness, diminish disintegration, and advance biodiversity. These practices add to better environments as well as result in stronger and useful horticultural frameworks. Furthermore, practical agribusiness underlines the utilization of natural and normal manures, diminishing the dependence on manufactured synthetic compounds that can destructively affect the climate and human wellbeing.

The idea of supportable horticulture stretches out past the field to incorporate the whole food inventory network. Neighborhood and natural food developments are picking up speed, empowering shoppers to help ranchers who focus on reasonable and harmless to the ecosystem rehearses. By picking privately obtained and natural items, purchasers add to decreasing the carbon impression related with food transportation and advancing practices that are less destructive to the climate.

In the domain of energy, maintainable practices are pivotal for lessening reliance on petroleum derivatives and moderating the effects of environmental change. The progress to environmentally friendly power sources, for example, sunlight based, wind, and hydropower, is a vital part of feasible energy rehearses. Dissimilar to petroleum products, sustainable power sources create power without delivering ozone harming substance emanations, which are significant supporters of an Earth-wide temperature boost.

Sun powered chargers, for instance, saddle energy from the sun and convert it into power, giving a perfect and sustainable power source. Wind turbines produce power by outfitting the dynamic energy of the breeze, and hydropower uses the energy of streaming water to create power.

By putting resources into and advancing the utilization of these inexhaustible innovations, social orders can fundamentally lessen their carbon impression and move towards a more economical energy future.

Energy proficiency is one more urgent part of manageable practices. By working on the proficiency of structures, machines, and modern cycles, we can diminish in general energy utilization and limit squander. This includes consolidating energy-effective advancements, carrying out better protection and plan in structures, and taking on rehearses that focus on asset preservation.

Transportation is an area where manageable practices can have a significant effect. The shift to electric vehicles, public transportation, and dynamic transportation modes, for example, strolling and cycling adds to lessening air contamination and diminishing reliance on petroleum products. The advancement of foundation that upholds these supportable methods of transportation, like bicycle paths and charging stations for electric vehicles, further energizes harmless to the ecosystem decisions.

Squander the board is a basic part of feasible practices. Conventional garbage removal techniques, like landfills and cremation, can adversely affect the climate, including soil and water contamination and the arrival of destructive ozone harming substances. Feasible waste administration includes lessening, reusing, and reusing materials to limit how much waste shipped off landfills.

Treating the soil is a viable practice that changes over natural waste into supplement rich soil corrections, lessening the requirement for manufactured composts and shutting the circle on supplement cycles. Furthermore, drives that advance stretched out maker obligation urge organizations to get a sense of ownership with the whole life pattern of their items, from creation to removal, encouraging a more reasonable way to deal with utilization.

Water preservation is a basic part of maintainable practices, given the rising weight on water assets around the world. Farming, industry, and homegrown exercises all add to water utilization and contamination. Feasible water the board includes carrying out rehearses that focus on water productivity, diminish contamination, and safeguard sea-going biological systems.

Dribble water system, water gathering, and water reusing are instances of manageable water rehearses in horticulture. Ventures can take on water-productive advancements, and people can contribute by utilizing water-saving machines, fixing spills, and rehearsing careful water utilization. Preservation endeavors additionally reach out to safeguarding regular water sources, like wetlands and watersheds, to keep up with biodiversity and biological system wellbeing.

Biodiversity protection is at the core of reasonable works on, perceiving the interconnectedness of every single living organic entity and their surroundings. Loss of biodiversity, driven by territory obliteration, contamination, environmental change, and overexploitation, represents an extreme danger to biological systems and their capacity to offer fundamental types of assistance.

Safeguarded regions, reforestation ventures, and natural surroundings reclamation drives are fundamental parts of biodiversity protection. Feasible ranger service rehearses, like particular logging and agroforestry, assist with keeping up with sound backwoods environments while giving significant assets. Furthermore, endeavors to battle unlawful natural life exchange and safeguard jeopardized species add to saving biodiversity and guaranteeing the equilibrium of environments.

Economical practices likewise reach out to the domain of metropolitan preparation and plan. Making bearable and strong urban communities includes coordinating green spaces, advancing energy-effective structures, and creating productive public transportation frameworks. Metropolitan agribusiness, roof gardens, and the utilization of economical materials in development add to the general maintainability of metropolitan conditions.

Natural training and mindfulness are crucial in advancing economical practices. By encouraging a comprehension of biological standards, asset preservation, and the effect of human exercises on the climate, social orders can settle on informed choices that focus on maintainability. Instructive drives at different levels, from schools to local area programs, assume a urgent part in molding a manageable mentality.

Government strategies and guidelines are instrumental in driving reasonable practices on a more extensive scale. Motivators for environmentally friendly power reception, guidelines on discharges and contamination, and the foundation of safeguarded regions are instances of strategy estimates that advance manageability. Public-private organizations and coordinated efforts between state run administrations, organizations, and common society further enhance the effect of practical drives.

Corporate obligation and maintainability revealing have acquired unmistakable quality as organizations perceive the significance of coordinating ecological, social, and administration (ESG) factors into their tasks. Economical strategic approaches go past benefit having to think about their effect on the climate and society. This incorporates lessening fossil fuel byproducts, embracing moral store network practices, and putting resources into social and local area advancement.

The round economy is an arising idea that lines up with economical practices by underscoring the decrease of waste and the productive utilization of assets. In contrast to the conventional direct economy, where items are fabricated, utilized, and discarded, the round economy advances methodologies like reusing, reusing, and revamping to expand the existence pattern of items.

All in all, manageable practices envelop a wide scope of procedures pointed toward safeguarding the climate, advancing social value, and guaranteeing monetary reasonability. From maintainable farming and environmentally friendly power to squander the board and biodiversity preservation, these practices address the interconnected difficulties presented by human exercises.

It isn't just a moral decision yet in addition a logical one to Embrace and advancing economical practices. As we face worldwide difficulties, for example, environmental change, asset exhaustion, and loss of biodiversity, coordinating supportability into our regular routines, organizations, and strategies becomes basic for a tough and agreeable future. By settling on cognizant decisions and embracing maintainable practices, we add to the prosperity of the planet and make ready for an additional manageable and impartial world.

6.3 Connecting with nature through avocado cultivation

Developing avocados at home gives an interesting and remunerating a potential open door to interface with nature on an individual level. Avocado trees (Persea Yankee folklore) are not just a wellspring of flavorful and nutritious organic product yet additionally a living connect to the regular world. The most common way of sustaining a little seed into a flourishing tree includes a more profound comprehension of vegetation, environment elements, and the interconnectedness of every living thing. Associating with nature through avocado development permits people to see the value in the patterns of development, find out about economical practices, and partake in the substantial their rewards for all the hard work.

The excursion starts with choosing a sound and ready avocado, from which the seed, or pit, will be extricated. This straightforward demonstration makes way for an intriguing course of germination and development. The avocado pit, once cleaned and ready, turns into the point of convergence of an excursion that traverses long stretches of time, at last prompting the development of a youthful avocado tree.

The germination cycle frequently includes suspending the avocado pit over a glass of water utilizing toothpicks. This basic arrangement permits the lower part of the pit to be lowered in water, establishing a climate helpful for root advancement. Persistence is key during this stage, as roots step by step stretch out from the pit, flagging the inception of the tree's development. Not all pits may effectively develop, underlining the requirement for different endeavors to build the odds of coming out on top.

When the roots have arrived at an adequate length, the sprouted pit is fit to be moved to soil. Choosing a well-depleting preparing blend and establishing the pit with the sharp end looking vertical are urgent moves toward giving the ideal circumstances to the youthful tree. As the avocado seedling arises, sensitive leaves spread out, denoting the start of an exceptional excursion toward development.

Avocado trees, local to tropical and subtropical districts, flourish in full daylight. Understanding the tree's light necessities is fundamental for its wellbeing and efficiency. For those developing avocados inside, putting the tree close to a south-bound window guarantees openness to sufficient daylight. The progressive acclimation of the tree to daylight is a critical stage, forestalling pressure and advancing vigorous development.

Watering is a crucial part of avocado tree care. While avocados favor reliably damp soil, overwatering can prompt root decay — a typical test in plant development. Finding some kind of harmony is fundamental, and this includes normal observing of soil dampness. As the tree develops, its water needs might advance, requiring changes in watering recurrence and volume.

Treating your avocado tree is one more basic part of care, especially for compartment developed trees. Picking a decent compost with a balance of nitrogen, phosphorus, and potassium upholds sound development. Applying compost as indicated by the producer's suggestions forestalls over-preparation and potential soil lopsided characteristics.

Avocado trees are weighty feeders, and appropriate nourishment adds to their general prosperity.

Pruning assumes a part in molding the avocado tree and advancing ideal development. Normal pruning keeps a reasonable size, empowers stretching, and dispenses with dead or harmed development. Be that as it may, a fragile equilibrium should be struck, as unnecessary pruning can pressure the tree. Cautious perception of the tree's regular structure directs the pruning system, guaranteeing an amicable and solid construction.

As the avocado tree develops, it will definitely enter the blooming stage, denoting the expected beginning of organic product creation. Avocado trees show a novel quality of having both male and female blossoms on a similar tree. Regardless of this, normal fertilization may not happen promptly. Presenting pollinators, like honey bees, or having numerous avocado trees can improve the probability of natural product advancement.

Persistence turns into a goodness as avocado trees find opportunity to develop and prove to be fruitful. The holding up period can differ, for certain trees creating organic product inside a couple of years and others taking more time. The elements impacting natural product improvement incorporate the tree's age, wellbeing, developing circumstances, and the adequacy of fertilization. The expectation and possible reap of local avocados become a demonstration of the commitment and care put resources into the development interaction.

Past the commonsense parts of avocado development lies a more profound association with nature. Growing an avocado tree turns into an excursion of revelation, permitting people to observe the complicated dance of life in the normal world. Noticing the rise of roots, the spreading out of leaves, and the improvement of blossoms cultivates a feeling of marvel and appreciation for the innate magnificence of vegetation.

The ecological advantages of developing avocados at home reach out past the singular tree. The act of reasonable and careful planting adds to a better biological system. Avocado trees, similar to all plants, assume an essential part in carbon sequestration, relieving the effects of environmental change. Their capacity to ingest carbon dioxide and delivery oxygen is an important natural help that upholds a decent and reasonable climate.

Moreover, avocados offer a chance to investigate maintainable and natural planting rehearses. Staying away from engineered pesticides and manures for normal options limits the natural effect of home cultivating. Friend planting, which includes decisively setting plants to help each other's development and discourage bothers, is a practical methodology that lines up with the standards of permaculture.

Developing avocados gives a substantial association with the food we eat. In a world overwhelmed by large scale manufacturing and worldwide stockpile chains, developing one's food offers a reviving other option. Local avocados not just add to a more maintainable and limited food framework yet in addition empower people to relish the kind of newly gathered organic product, liberated from the calculated intricacies of transportation and capacity.

The demonstration of developing avocados turns into a microcosm of manageable living. The comprehension of water preservation, soil wellbeing, and the sensitive equilibrium of biological systems acquired through avocado development can be applied to more extensive ecological stewardship. Avocado trees, with their rich green foliage and velvety natural products, act as ministers of maintainable practices inside the bounds of one's home.

As people leave on the excursion of avocado development, they become piece of a bigger development upholding for a nearer relationship with nature. The demonstration of sustaining a living creature from seed to development imparts a feeling of obligation and care for the climate. This association reaches out past the limits of the nursery, impacting way of life decisions and encouraging a more profound appreciation for the Earth and its environments.

The advantages of associating with nature through avocado development are not restricted to the ecological domain. Developing avocados gives a helpful and careful experience that adds to in general prosperity.

The demonstration of keeping an eye on a residing creature, noticing its development, and receiving the benefits of local natural product lines up with rehearses known to decrease pressure, advance emotional wellness, and improve a feeling of satisfaction.

Avocado development likewise fills in as a door to more extensive discussions about supportability and natural cognizance. Imparting the experience to companions, family, or local area individuals makes an expanding influence, motivating others to investigate their association with nature. Local area nurseries, studios, and instructive drives revolved around supportable practices further intensify the effect of avocado development as an impetus for positive change.

All in all, interfacing with nature through avocado development is a multi-layered venture that rises above the limits of cultivation. It is a chance to observe the wonders of vegetation, embrace reasonable practices, and relish the one's rewards for all the hard work. Avocado trees, with their rich foliage and smooth natural products, act as diplomats of the regular world inside the personal setting of a nursery or living space.

The course of avocado development welcomes people to become stewards of the climate, cultivating a feeling of obligation and care for the planet. As avocados develop from seeds to thriving trees, they become images of flexibility, persistence, and the interconnectedness of every single living thing. Past the unmistakable advantages of local organic product, avocado development offers a pathway to a more economical and agreeable relationship with nature — one that leaves an enduring effect on people, networks, and the actual Earth.

Developing avocados at home offers a one of a kind and compensating an open door to interface with nature on an individual level. Avocado trees (Persea History of the U.S) yield delectable and nutritious organic product as well as give a living connect to the normal world. The most common way of sustaining a little seed into a flourishing tree includes a more profound comprehension of vegetation, environment elements, and the interconnectedness of every living thing. Associating with nature through avocado development permits people to see the value in the patterns of development, find out about supportable practices, and partake in the unmistakable their rewards for all the hard work.

The excursion starts with the determination of a sound and ready avocado, from which the seed or pit will be separated. This straightforward demonstration makes way for an entrancing course of germination and development. The avocado pit, once cleaned and ready, turns into the point of convergence of an excursion that traverses long stretches of time, eventually prompting the development of a youthful avocado tree.

Germination frequently includes suspending the avocado pit over a glass of water utilizing toothpicks. This arrangement permits the lower part of the pit to be lowered in water, establishing a climate helpful for root advancement. Persistence is key during this stage, as roots step by step reach out from the pit, flagging the commencement of the tree's development. Not all pits may effectively sprout, underlining the requirement for different endeavors to build the odds of coming out on top.

When the roots have arrived at an adequate length, the sprouted pit is fit to be moved to soil. Picking a well-depleting preparing blend and establishing the pit with the sharp end looking vertical are essential moves toward giving the ideal circumstances to the youthful tree. As the avocado seedling arises, sensitive leaves spread out, denoting the start of a wonderful excursion toward development.

Avocado trees, local to tropical and subtropical districts, flourish in full daylight. Understanding the tree's light necessities is fundamental for its wellbeing and efficiency. For those developing avocados inside, setting the tree close to a south-bound window guarantees openness to sufficient daylight. The progressive acclimation of the tree to daylight is a vital stage, forestalling pressure and advancing vigorous development.

Watering is a major part of avocado tree care. While avocados favor reliably damp soil, overwatering can prompt root decay — a typical test in plant development. Finding some kind of harmony is fundamental, and this includes ordinary checking of soil dampness. As the tree develops, its water needs might advance, requiring changes in watering recurrence and volume.

Preparing your avocado tree is one more basic part of care, especially for holder developed trees. Picking a fair compost with a balance of nitrogen, phosphorus, and potassium upholds sound development. Applying manure as indicated by the maker's suggestions forestalls over-treatment and potential soil lopsided characteristics. Avocado trees are weighty feeders, and appropriate sustenance adds to their general prosperity.

Pruning assumes a part in molding the avocado tree and advancing ideal development. Normal pruning keeps a reasonable size, supports fanning, and disposes of dead or harmed development. In any case, a fragile equilibrium should be struck, as unnecessary pruning can pressure the tree. Cautious perception of the tree's regular structure directs the pruning system, guaranteeing an agreeable and sound design.

As the avocado tree develops, it will definitely enter the blooming stage, denoting the likely beginning of natural product creation. Avocado trees show a special trait of having both male and female blossoms on a similar tree. In spite of this, regular fertilization may not happen promptly. Presenting pollinators, like honey bees, or having different avocado trees can improve the probability of natural product advancement.

Persistence turns into a goodness as avocado trees carve out opportunity to develop and prove to be fruitful. The holding up period can shift, for certain trees delivering natural product inside a couple of years and others taking more time. The variables affecting organic product advancement incorporate the tree's age, wellbeing, developing circumstances, and the adequacy of fertilization. The expectation and possible collect of local avocados become a demonstration of the devotion and care put resources into the development interaction.

Past the viable parts of avocado development lies a more profound association with nature. Growing an avocado tree turns into an excursion of revelation, permitting people to observe the unpredictable dance of life in the normal world. Noticing the rise of roots, the spreading out of leaves, and the improvement of blossoms cultivates a feeling of miracle and appreciation for the intrinsic magnificence of vegetation.

The natural advantages of developing avocados at home reach out past the singular tree. The act of economical and careful planting adds to a better biological system. Avocado trees, similar to all plants, assume a critical part in carbon sequestration, relieving the effects of environmental change. Their capacity to retain carbon dioxide and delivery oxygen is a significant biological help that upholds a fair and manageable climate.

Moreover, avocados offer a chance to investigate supportable and natural cultivating rehearses. Staying away from manufactured pesticides and composts for regular choices limits the ecological effect of home cultivating. Friend planting, which includes decisively putting plants to help each other's development and deflect bothers, is a reasonable methodology that lines up with the standards of permaculture.

Developing avocados gives an unmistakable association with the food we devour. In a world overwhelmed by large scale manufacturing and worldwide stock chains, developing one's food offers a reviving other option. Local avocados not just add to a more economical and limited food framework yet in addition empower people to relish the kind of newly collected natural product, liberated from the strategic intricacies of transportation and capacity.

The demonstration of developing avocados turns into a microcosm of economical living. The comprehension of water preservation, soil wellbeing, and the fragile equilibrium of biological systems acquired through avocado development can be applied to more extensive natural stewardship. Avocado trees, with their rich green foliage and smooth organic products, act as envoys of maintainable practices inside the bounds of one's home.

As people set out on the excursion of avocado development, they become piece of a bigger development upholding for a nearer relationship with nature. The demonstration of sustaining a living organic entity from seed to development ingrains a feeling of obligation and care for the climate. This association stretches out past the limits of the nursery, impacting way of life decisions and encouraging a more profound appreciation for the Earth and its environments.

The advantages of interfacing with nature through avocado development are not restricted to the ecological domain. Developing avocados gives a restorative and careful experience that adds to by and large prosperity. The demonstration of watching out professionally life form, noticing its development, and receiving the benefits of local natural product lines up with rehearses known to diminish pressure, advance emotional wellness, and improve a feeling of satisfaction.

Avocado development likewise fills in as a passage to more extensive discussions about maintainability and natural cognizance. Offering the experience to companions, family, or local area individuals makes a gradually expanding influence, motivating others to investigate their association with nature.

Local area nurseries, studios, and instructive drives revolved around economical practices further intensify the effect of avocado development as an impetus for positive change.

8

Chapter 7

Avocado Lifestyle: Nurturing Body and Soul

In the clamoring embroidery of contemporary presence, where the requests of a speedy world frequently appear to infringe upon the limits of individual prosperity, the idea of an all encompassing way of life has arisen as a directing reference point for some. Among the horde of ways to deal with prosperity, the Avocado Way of life stands apart as a worldview that interweaves the supporting of both body and soul. This way of life, established in a significant comprehension of the interconnectedness of physical and emotional well-being, has gathered consideration for its accentuation on care, nourishment, and manageable practices.

At the core of the Avocado Way of life is the acknowledgment that the psyche and body are inseparably connected, impacting and molding each other in a sensitive dance. In a world that frequently compartmentalizes wellbeing into physical and mental spaces, this comprehensive methodology looks to overcome any issues between the two, perceiving that genuine prosperity rises up out of an agreeable collaboration among body and soul.

Care, a foundation of the Avocado Way of life, offers a vital pathway towards accomplishing this congruity. In a culture that frequently extols performing various tasks and ceaseless hecticness, care fills in as a contradiction — a training that urges people to secure themselves right now. Whether through reflection, profound breathing activities, or other pensive practices, care turns into a device for developing mindfulness and encouraging a feeling of inward equilibrium.

The Avocado Way of life broadens this care past individual prosperity and integrates it into the texture of day to day living. It urges people to be available in their inside scenes as well as in their collaborations with the outer world. This mindfulness, when applied to sustenance, changes the demonstration of eating into a careful custom — one that commends the sustenance of the body and the delight of relishing each nibble.

Nourishment, one more major mainstay of the Avocado Way of life, becomes the overwhelming focus for the purpose of cultivating actual wellbeing and imperativeness. The avocado, a flexible and supplement rich organic product, turns into an image of this wholesome concentration. Loaded with heart-sound monounsaturated fats, nutrients, and minerals, avocados offer a healthy starting point for a reasonable eating routine.

The Avocado Way of life stresses a plant-based, entire food sources way to deal with sustenance, perceiving the significant effect of dietary decisions on both individual wellbeing and the more extensive natural scene. This approach lines up with the standards of supportability, asking people to think about the natural impression of their food decisions. From supporting nearby ranchers to decreasing food squander, the Avocado Way of life advocate an all encompassing comprehension of nourishment that rises above simple food.

Manageability, a center precept of the Avocado Way of life, stretches out past dietary contemplations to include a more extensive natural cognizance. The way of life urges people to take on rehearses that limit their natural effect, perceiving the interconnectedness of all life on The planet. This might include lessening single-utilize plastic utilization, embracing sustainable power sources, or partaking in local area drives pointed toward saving the regular world.

In the domain of active work, the Avocado Way of life advocates for development that goes past the bounds of customary activity. While organized exercises have their place, the way of life urges people to participate in exercises that give pleasure and satisfaction — whether it be moving, climbing, or rehearsing yoga. This point of view on actual work rises above the idea of activity as a simple commitment and on second thought outlines it as a festival of the body's capacities.

The Avocado Way of life's comprehensive way to deal with prosperity incorporates the person as well as the local area. It perceives the significance of social associations in encouraging a feeling of having a place and backing.

Whether through shared dinners, collective social occasions, or cooperative tasks, the way of life urges people to wind around an embroidery of significant connections that add to a feeling of common perspective and interconnectedness.

Key to the Avocado Way of life is the possibility that taking care of oneself is definitely not a narrow minded extravagance however a crucial need. In a world that frequently extols exhaust and ceaseless efficiency, the way of life welcomes people to focus on their prosperity without culpability. This might include defining limits, developing serene practices, or essentially taking snapshots of interruption in the midst of life's requests.

The Avocado Way of life additionally perceives the job of imagination in sustaining the spirit. Whether communicated through craftsmanship, composing, music, or different structures, inventiveness turns into a method for taking advantage of the inward supplies of motivation and self-articulation. In a general public that frequently esteems efficiency over imagination, this part of the way of life fills in as a sign of the natural worth of creative undertakings in enhancing the human experience.

As the Avocado Way of life unfurls as an embroidery woven from care, sustenance, manageability, actual work, local area, taking care of oneself, and innovativeness, it welcomes people to leave on an excursion of self-revelation and development. It challenges ordinary ideas of progress and joy, empowering a reexamination of needs for a more adjusted and satisfying presence.

In the domain of care, the Avocado Way of life draws motivation from antiquated thoughtful customs while adjusting to the requests of present day life. Care rehearses, whether established in contemplation, careful eating, or different structures, become devices for exploring the intricacies of the brain and developing a feeling of presence. In a world set apart by steady interruptions and data over-burden, care arises as a safe-haven — a space where people can reconnect with themselves and their general surroundings.

Sustenance, as a point of convergence of the Avocado Way of life, goes past the regular standards of slimming down and limitation. It embraces a way of thinking of overflow, praising the different exhibit of supplement thick food sources that add to generally prosperity. The avocado, with its velvety surface and rich flavor, turns into an image of this overflow — a flexible fixing that adds healthy benefit as well as a hint of extravagance to dinners.

The Avocado Way of life's obligation to maintainability mirrors a consciousness of the critical need to address ecological difficulties. It perceives that singular decisions, regardless of how apparently little, on the whole add to the bigger natural picture. By taking on rehearses that focus on the strength of the planet, the way of life supports a shift towards a more economical and regenerative approach to everyday life.

In the domain of actual work, the Avocado Way of life commends the variety of development and urges people to track down happiness in being dynamic. From the delicate progression of yoga to the elation of dance, actual work turns into a method for communicating the body's imperativeness and reconnecting with the intrinsic joy of development. This viewpoint on practice rises above the limited bounds of wellness objectives and embraces a more comprehensive perspective on the body's capacities.

Local area, as a necessary part of the Avocado Way of life, underlines the interconnectedness of people inside a more extensive social setting. The way of life energizes the development of significant connections and the formation of strong networks that encourage a feeling of having a place. In a world that frequently underscores individual accomplishment, the Avocado Way of life perceives the significance of shared encounters and cooperative undertakings in building a feeling of aggregate prosperity.

Taking care of oneself, a foundation of the Avocado Way of life, challenges the idea that hecticness is inseparable from efficiency. It welcomes people to focus on their psychological and close to home prosperity, perceiving that genuine efficiency emerges from a groundwork of internal equilibrium. This might include defining limits, expressing no to exorbitant requests, and embracing rehearses that recharge the soul.

Inventiveness, as a fundamental component of the Avocado Way of life, recognizes the extraordinary force of creative articulation. Whether through visual expressions, composing, or different types of inventiveness, people are urged to take advantage of their innovative limits and investigate the domains of self-articulation. In a world that frequently esteems logical reasoning, the way of life commends the one of a kind gifts of imagination in cultivating a feeling of marvel and association with the more profound flows of life.

As people embrace the Avocado Way of life, they set out on an excursion of self-revelation and taking care of oneself. A way welcomes thoughtfulness, requesting that people consider their qualities, needs, and the effect of their decisions on themselves and the world. The Avocado Way of life is certainly not an inflexible arrangement of rules yet an adaptable structure that adjusts to the different requirements and conditions of people.

In the domain of care, the Avocado Way of life welcomes people to develop a day to day practice of presence. This might include reflection, careful breathing, or basically stopping to relish the extravagance of every second. As people coordinate care into their lives, they become more sensitive to the unobtrusive subtleties of their viewpoints, feelings, and actual sensations.

Nourishment, as a critical part of the Avocado Way of life, urges people to move toward eating with appreciation and mindfulness. The demonstration of getting ready and devouring food turns into a careful custom, a valuable chance to feed the body and value the interconnected snare of life that supports us.

The avocado, with its energetic green tints and smooth surface, turns into an image of this careful way to deal with sustenance — a suggestion to enjoy the kinds of the current second.

Manageability, profoundly imbued in the Avocado Way of life, prompts people to think about the natural effect of their decisions. From decreasing waste to supporting eco-accommodating drives, the way of life empowers a shift towards cognizant utilization. As people adjust their activities to environmental standards, they become stewards of the planet, adding to the prosperity of the Earth and people in the future.

In the domain of actual work, the Avocado Way of life advocates for an upbeat and natural way to deal with development. As opposed to survey practice as a task, people are urged to investigate exercises that give joy and essentialness. Whether it's a relaxed stroll in nature or an unconstrained dance in the lounge room, development turns into an outflow of the body's inborn insight and a festival of life.

Local area, as a fundamental component of the Avocado Way of life, accentuates the interconnectedness of people inside the bigger snare of society. The way of life energizes the development of significant connections, encouraging a feeling of mutual perspective and backing. In a world that frequently complements independence, the Avocado Way of life perceives the force of local area in sustaining a feeling of having a place and aggregate prosperity.

Taking care of oneself, woven into the texture of the Avocado Way of life, challenges the overall story that consistent efficiency is the proportion of achievement. The way of life urges people to focus on rest, revival, and exercises that give pleasure. As people embrace taking care of oneself, they renew their own stores as well as add to a culture that values prosperity over unending hecticness.

Imagination, as a directing power in the Avocado Way of life, welcomes people to investigate the endless domains of self-articulation. Whether through visual expressions, composing, or other inventive pursuits, people tap into the wellspring of their creative mind. Innovativeness turns into an instrument for self-disclosure, a method for rising above constraints, and a wellspring of motivation that mixes existence with magnificence and significance.

As the Avocado Way of life turns into a lived insight, people end up on a groundbreaking excursion — one that rises above the limits of traditional standards and welcomes a reexamination of needs. An excursion respects the interconnectedness of all parts of life, perceiving the significant effect of careful decisions on private prosperity and the prosperity of the planet.

In the embroidery of the Avocado Way of life, each string addresses a feature of an all encompassing presence. Care, sustenance, maintainability, actual work, local area, taking care of oneself, and innovativeness wind around together to make a dynamic and amicable approach to everyday life. The way of life is definitely not an unbending solution however an adaptable and versatile system that develops with the interesting necessities and conditions of people.

In the domain of care, the Avocado Way of life turns into a safehaven for the brain. People develop an act of mindfulness that stretches out past the limits of formal contemplation to pervade each part of their lives. This care isn't tied in with getting away from the difficulties of life however turning around them with serenity, answering with lucidity and empathy.

Nourishment, as a focal mainstay of the Avocado Way of life, welcomes people to move toward food with veneration. The demonstration of eating turns into a consecrated custom — a fellowship with the Earth and a festival of the interconnected trap of life. The avocado, with its delectable taste and feeding properties, encapsulates the way of thinking of overflow and appreciation that describes this way to deal with sustenance.

Manageability, profoundly imbued in the Avocado Way of life, stretches out past individual decisions to a more extensive biological viewpoint. It prompts people to consider the drawn out results of their activities and settle on decisions that line up with the wellbeing of the planet. The way of life encourages a feeling of obligation, asking people to become cognizant stewards of the Earth.

In the domain of active work, the Avocado Way of life praises the variety of development. People are urged to track down happiness in being dynamic, whether through organized exercises or unconstrained articulations of imperativeness. The accentuation is on developing a relationship with the body that is established in joy and appreciation for its capacities.

Local area, as a fundamental component of the Avocado Way of life, accentuates the significance of human association. People are welcome to fabricate connections that go past surface collaborations, cultivating a feeling of having a place and backing. The way of life perceives the force of local area in enhancing individual prosperity and adding to an aggregate feeling of direction.

Taking care of oneself, intertwined with the texture of the Avocado Way of life, challenges the thought that consistent efficiency is the way to satisfaction. It welcomes people to stand by listening to their own requirements, focus on rest, and participate in exercises that feed the spirit. Taking care of oneself turns into an extreme demonstration of insubordination to a culture that frequently ignores the significance of prosperity.

Imagination, as a directing power in the Avocado Way of life, welcomes people to investigate the boundless domains of creative mind. Whether through imaginative undertakings or inventive critical thinking, innovativeness turns into a method for self-articulation and association with the more profound flows of life. The way of life praises the one of a kind gifts of every person and energizes the declaration of imagination in the entirety of its structures.

As people submerge themselves in the Avocado Way of life, they become planners of their own prosperity. The way of life isn't an objective yet a continuous excursion — an excursion that unfurls in the everyday decisions, practices, and connections that shape one's presence. An excursion welcomes people to recover office over their lives and adjust their activities to their most profound qualities.

In the domain of care, the Avocado Way of life is a call to presence — a call to possess every second with full mindfulness. Whether through proper contemplation rehearses or casual snapshots of care, people develop a condition of increased cognizance that imbues each part of their lives. This care turns into a compass, directing people through the intricacies of the cutting edge world.

Sustenance, as a foundation of the Avocado Way of life, is a festival of the World's abundance. The way of life urges people to enjoy the kinds of entire, plant-based food varieties and value the interconnected snare of life that supports us. The avocado, with its velvety surface and dynamic green shades, turns into an image of this plentiful and sustaining way to deal with eating.

Maintainability, well established in the Avocado Way of life, is a promise to the prosperity of the planet. It prompts people to think about the natural effect of their decisions and embrace rehearses that add to biological concordance. The way of life encourages a feeling of environmental citizenship, welcoming people to become careful caretakers of the Earth.

In the domain of active work, the Avocado Way of life is an encouragement to move with satisfaction and aim. As opposed to survey practice as a task, people are urged to investigate exercises that give joy and essentialness. The accentuation is on developing a relationship with the body that is set apart by appreciation and regard for its capacities.

Local area, as a basic part of the Avocado Way of life, is an acknowledgment of the reliance of living souls. The way of life urges people to construct significant associations, encouraging.

7.1 The holistic approach to health and well-being

The all encompassing way to deal with wellbeing and prosperity is an extensive viewpoint that thinks about the interconnectedness of different parts of a singular's life. It goes past the customary spotlight on actual wellbeing and integrates mental, close to home, social, and profound aspects. This comprehensive model perceives that these aspects are related, impacting each other and all in all adding to an individual's general prosperity.

Actual wellbeing is a crucial part of the all encompassing methodology. It includes the well-working of the body's frameworks, including cardiovascular, respiratory, stomach related, and outer muscle frameworks. Standard activity, a fair eating routine, adequate rest, and legitimate hydration are key variables in keeping up with actual wellbeing. Moreover, preventive measures, for example, immunizations and screenings assume a critical part in early location and the executives of potential medical problems.

Emotional wellness is one more basic component of comprehensive prosperity. It incorporates mental capabilities, close to home soundness, and mental flexibility. Psychological well-being difficulties, like tension and gloom, can essentially influence an individual's general prosperity. All encompassing ways to deal with psychological wellness include remedial intercessions, guiding, and procedures for stress the board. Care practices, reflection, and mental conduct treatment are frequently integrated to improve mental prosperity.

Profound prosperity is firmly associated with psychological well-being and includes the capacity to grasp, express, and deal with one's feelings. Building the capacity to understand people on a deeper level is a critical part of the all encompassing methodology, as it empowers people to really explore relational connections. Social help, relational abilities, and mindfulness add to profound prosperity. Developing solid connections and communicating feelings in a helpful way are fundamental for keeping up with close to home equilibrium.

The social element of prosperity underscores the effect of connections, local area, and cultural associations on a singular's wellbeing. People are intrinsically friendly creatures, and the nature of social cooperations significantly affects by and large prosperity. Solid social associations offer profound help, diminish sensations of seclusion, and add to a feeling of having a place. Constructing and keeping up with solid associations with family, companions, and local area individuals are essential to the comprehensive way to deal with prosperity.

Otherworldly prosperity incorporates a feeling of direction, importance, and association with an option that could be more significant than oneself. It doesn't be guaranteed to must be attached to a particular strict conviction yet includes a more profound investigation of one's qualities, convictions, and existential inquiries. For some's purposes, otherworldliness might include coordinated religion, while for other people, it might appear through nature, workmanship, or individual reflection. Supporting profound prosperity frequently includes practices like contemplation, petition, or participating in exercises that line up with one's qualities.

The comprehensive way to deal with wellbeing and prosperity perceives the perplexing interaction between these aspects. Accomplishing equilibrium and congruity across physical, mental, profound, social, and otherworldly perspectives is a dynamic and progressing process. An unsettling influence in one aspect can have far reaching influences on others, featuring the significance of tending to wellbeing and prosperity comprehensively.

Preventive estimates assume a critical part in keeping up with by and large prosperity. Ordinary wellbeing check-ups, screenings, and inoculations are fundamental parts of preventive consideration. Early discovery of medical problems considers opportune mediation and the executives, forestalling the heightening of issues. Moreover, embracing a solid way of life that incorporates ordinary activity, a nutritious eating regimen, and stress the board adds to forestalling different medical issue.

Sustenance is a foundation of comprehensive wellbeing, influencing both physical and mental prosperity. An even eating regimen gives fundamental supplements that help importantphysical processes and advance generally speaking wellbeing. The association among diet and emotional well-being is progressively perceived, with research proposing that specific supplements assume a part in temperament guideline and mental capability. Incorporating entire food varieties, organic products, vegetables, and satisfactory hydration into one's eating regimen is fundamental for all encompassing prosperity.

Practice isn't just useful for actual wellbeing yet in addition decidedly affects mental and close to home prosperity. Customary active work discharges endorphins, which are synapses that add to sensations of satisfaction and decrease pressure. Practice is additionally connected to worked on mental capability and better rest quality. Consolidating a blend of high-impact, strength, and adaptability practices into a normal improves in general wellness and supports all encompassing prosperity.

Rest is a central part of physical and emotional wellness. Quality rest is fundamental for the body's recuperation, insusceptible capability, and mental cycles. Ongoing lack of sleep is related with an expanded gamble of different ailments, including cardiovascular infection, diabetes, and emotional wellness problems. Creating sound rest propensities, for example, keeping a reliable rest plan and establishing a helpful rest climate, is significant for all encompassing prosperity.

Stress the executives is a vital part of the all encompassing methodology, given the inescapable effect of weight on wellbeing. Constant pressure is connected to different medical problems, including cardiovascular issues, stomach related messes, and compromised insusceptible capability. Comprehensive pressure the executives includes embracing methods like care, reflection, profound breathing activities, and moderate muscle unwinding. Coordinating these practices into day to day existence upholds generally speaking prosperity by advancing unwinding and strength notwithstanding stressors.

Emotional well-being mindfulness and destigmatization are fundamental parts of the all encompassing methodology. Perceiving the significance of mental prosperity and understanding that psychological wellness challenges are normal human encounters add to establishing a steady climate.

Open correspondence, training, and admittance to emotional well-being assets are vital for tending to emotional wellness issues extensively. Coordinating emotional well-being into generally medical care guarantees an all encompassing methodology that thinks about both physical and mental perspectives.

All encompassing medical care stretches out past conventional clinical mediations to embrace integral and elective treatments. Integrative medication consolidates ordinary clinical practices with proof based correlative treatments. Modalities, for example, needle therapy, chiropractic care, natural medication, and back rub treatment are instances of approaches that might be coordinated into comprehensive medical services. The objective is to address the person in general, considering physical, mental, and close to home viewpoints in treatment plans.

Developing care is a focal subject in the all encompassing way to deal with prosperity. Care includes focusing on the current second without judgment. Practices like care contemplation, yoga, and jujitsu advance mindfulness and presence. Research proposes that care can diminish pressure, work on mental lucidity, and improve generally personal satisfaction. Integrating care into everyday schedules encourages a more profound association with one's encounters and supports all encompassing prosperity.

Ecological prosperity is a frequently disregarded element of all encompassing wellbeing. The nature of the climate wherein people live and work can influence their general prosperity. Natural factors, for example, air and water quality, admittance to green spaces, and openness to poisons can impact wellbeing results. Advancing economical works on, upholding for natural equity, and interfacing with nature add to comprehensive prosperity by thinking about the more extensive environmental setting.

Comprehensive schooling assumes a part in encouraging an outlook that qualities and focuses on by and large prosperity. School systems that consolidate all encompassing methodologies center around scholastic accomplishment as well as on the improvement of social, profound, and fundamental abilities. Incorporating care rehearses, actual training, and emotional well-being instruction into school educational plans adds to the all encompassing improvement of people since early on.

Work environment prosperity is a critical part of the all encompassing methodology, given how much time people spend in proficient conditions. Making work areas that focus on physical and emotional wellness cultivates representative fulfillment and efficiency. Practices, for example, adaptable plans for getting work done, stress decrease projects, and drives that advance balance between fun and serious activities add to comprehensive prosperity in the working environment.

The job of local area and social help couldn't possibly be more significant in comprehensive prosperity. Building solid social associations, whether through family, companions, or local area associations, gives a feeling of having a place and basic reassurance. Social segregation is related with unfriendly wellbeing results, stressing the significance of local area commitment. Aggregate endeavors to resolve social issues, advance inclusivity, and backing weak populaces add to the general prosperity of society.

Social and variety contemplations are indispensable to the all encompassing methodology. Perceiving and regarding different points of view, values, and practices add to a more comprehensive comprehension of prosperity. Social capability in medical care guarantees that people get customized and socially touchy administrations. Embracing variety encourages an all encompassing methodology that recognizes the special requirements and encounters of various populaces.

Comprehensive prosperity is a continuous excursion that requires self-reflection and a promise to self-awareness. Practices, for example, journaling, taking care of oneself schedules, and defining purposeful objectives add to mindfulness and self-improvement. The capacity to adjust to life's difficulties, develop strength, and keep a positive outlook are fundamental parts of all encompassing prosperity.

The coordination of innovation into all encompassing medical care is a developing pattern. Portable applications, wearable gadgets, and telehealth administrations give instruments to people to follow and oversee different parts of their wellbeing. Innovation additionally works with admittance to data, assets, and encouraging groups of people. Incorporating innovation mindfully and morally into comprehensive medical services upgrades the availability and adequacy of prosperity rehearses.

Examination and proof based rehearses are fundamental for propelling the comprehension of all encompassing wellbeing. Proceeded with logical investigation into the interconnectedness of physical, mental, close to home, social, and profound aspects adds to the improvement of viable intercessions. Cooperative endeavors between scientists, medical services experts, and people are pivotal for advancing proof based comprehensive ways to deal with prosperity.

Strategy and promotion assume a basic part in supporting comprehensive prosperity at the cultural level. Upholding for strategies that focus on preventive consideration, psychological well-being administrations, and ecological manageability adds to a comprehensive methodology in medical services. Tending to social determinants of wellbeing, like pay disparity and admittance to instruction, is fundamental for making conditions that help the general prosperity of networks.

7.2 Building a balanced lifestyle with avocados at its core

Building a reasonable way of life is a diverse undertaking that includes integrating nutritious food sources, keeping up with active work, overseeing pressure, and encouraging positive propensities. Avocados, with their rich supplement profile and flexibility, can assume a focal part in supporting a reasonable and sound way of life. From giving fundamental supplements to offering culinary adaptability, avocados offer various advantages that add to in general prosperity.

Avocados are prestigious for their supplement thickness, containing various nutrients, minerals, and helpful mixtures. They are especially wealthy in monounsaturated fats, which are heart-solid fats related with worked on cardiovascular wellbeing. The monounsaturated fats in avocados, primarily oleic corrosive, have been connected to diminished irritation and lower levels of awful cholesterol (LDL) while expanding great cholesterol (HDL).

Past their solid fat substance, avocados are a decent wellspring of nutrients and minerals. They contain potassium, a fundamental mineral for keeping up with legitimate pulse levels, and are a fair wellspring of nutrients C, E, K, and B-6. Avocados likewise give folate, a significant supplement for cell division and DNA combination, making them an important expansion to a reasonable eating regimen.

Notwithstanding their wholesome substance, avocados offer dietary fiber, which upholds stomach related wellbeing and keeps a sensation of completion. The blend of solid fats and fiber creates avocados a satisfying food that can be helpful for weight the executives when included as a feature of a balanced eating regimen.

The flexibility of avocados makes them an important fixing in a large number of dishes. Whether cut on toast, mixed into a smoothie, added to plates of mixed greens, or utilized as a rich base for sauces and dressings, avocados upgrade the flavor and surface of different dinners. This culinary flexibility makes it simple to integrate avocados into a different and adjusted diet, taking care of various taste inclinations and dietary requirements.

A vital part of building a decent way of life is keeping up with legitimate piece control and being aware of by and large calorie consumption. While avocados give various medical advantages, consuming them in moderation is fundamental. Because of their caloric thickness, unnecessary admission might add to an overconsumption of calories. Adjusting the incorporation of avocados with other supplement thick food sources guarantees a balanced and calorie-proper eating routine.

Active work is a foundation of a fair way of life, and avocados can add to the dietary help required for a functioning body. The potassium in avocados assumes a part in muscle capability, making them an important nourishment for those taking part in normal activity.

Moreover, the sound fats in avocados act as a wellspring of supported energy, making them a helpful nibble choice for people driving a functioning way of life.

Overseeing pressure is one more urgent part of building a reasonable way of life. Persistent pressure can antagonistically affect both physical and mental prosperity. Avocados contain pressure alleviating supplements, for example, B nutrients, including B-6 and folate, which are associated with the combination of synapses that control temperament. The demonstration of planning and getting a charge out of avocado-based feasts can likewise act as a careful and stress-decreasing action.

Remembering avocados for a fair way of life lines up with more extensive dietary suggestions that underline entire, negligibly handled food varieties. This approach urges people to focus on supplement rich food sources while limiting the admission of profoundly handled and sweet choices. Avocados, in general food with an abundance of supplements, fit flawlessly into this dietary system.

The advantages of avocados stretch out past their nourishing substance to incorporate potential wellbeing advancing properties. A few examinations recommend that the bioactive mixtures tracked down in avocados, like carotenoids and tocopherols, may have cell reinforcement and mitigating impacts. These properties could add to decreasing the gamble of persistent infections and supporting in general wellbeing.

One of the remarkable highlights of avocados is their expected job in advancing solid skin. The blend of nutrients C and E, alongside monounsaturated fats, upholds skin wellbeing and hydration. Furthermore, avocados contain cell reinforcements that might assist with safeguarding the skin from the harming impacts of free extremists. Remembering avocados for a balanced eating routine can add to a comprehensive way to deal with skincare.

It's vital to take note of that singular dietary necessities differ, and a fair way of life includes thinking about private inclinations, wellbeing objectives, and a particular dietary limitations or conditions. While avocados offer a scope of advantages, people with explicit sensitivities or responsive qualities ought to be aware of their own wholesome necessities. Talking with a medical services proficient or an enrolled dietitian can give customized direction on integrating avocados into a fair eating routine.

With regards to building a decent way of life, the job of hydration ought not be ignored. While avocados add to by and large water admission, particularly when drunk in their normal express, focusing on satisfactory water utilization over the course of the day is fundamental. Remaining hydrated upholds different physical processes, including assimilation, supplement transport, and temperature guideline.

Building a reasonable way of life includes developing positive propensities past nourishment, including standard rest, stress the board, and care rehearses. Avocados, with their supplement rich profile, can supplement these way of life factors by giving fundamental supplements that help by and large wellbeing. The consideration of avocados in a reasonable eating regimen lines up with the more extensive idea of comprehensive prosperity, perceiving the interconnectedness of different way of life components.

In rundown, fabricating a fair way of life with avocados at its center includes an all encompassing way to deal with prosperity. Avocados add to generally wellbeing through their supplement thickness, solid fats, and flexibility in culinary applications. Remembering avocados for a balanced eating routine backings cardiovascular wellbeing, gives fundamental nutrients and minerals, and offers likely advantages for skin wellbeing.

Notwithstanding, balance is vital, and control is fundamental to forestall unnecessary calorie consumption. Active work, stress the executives, and other positive way of life propensities ought to likewise be viewed as chasing after generally speaking prosperity. Avocados can be a significant and charming part of a decent way of life, upgrading the nourishing nature of dinners and advancing comprehensive wellbeing.

7.3 Personal stories and testimonials of individuals who have embraced the avocado lifestyle

Individual stories and tributes frequently act as strong accounts that shed light on the genuine encounters of people who have embraced a specific way of life. On account of the avocado way of life, these accounts give experiences into what incorporating avocados into everyday sustenance has meant for individuals' wellbeing, prosperity, and in general personal satisfaction. Through an assortment of different stories, we can investigate the different ways people have integrated avocados into their eating regimens and the positive results they have seen.

One individual offers their excursion of finding the avocado as a groundbreaking expansion to their eating routine. Having battled with finding fulfilling and nutritious food sources, this individual coincidentally found the avocado and was flabbergasted by its flexibility and nourishing advantages. They depict how avocados turned into a staple in their feasts, supplanting less supplement thick choices. The sound fats in avocados gave supported energy, and the rich surface turned into a magnificent component in both flavorful and sweet dishes. This individual underlines how the presentation of avocados worked on their actual wellbeing as well as decidedly impacted their psychological prosperity, making a feeling of equilibrium and fulfillment in their dietary decisions.

Another individual story digs into the excursion of a wellness lover who perceived the worth of avocados in supporting their dynamic way of life. This individual underscores the potassium content in avocados, which assumes an essential part in muscle capability and recuperation.

They depict integrating avocados into pre-and post-exercise feasts, featuring the advantages of the supplement rich natural product in upgrading their actual exhibition. The flexibility of avocados in different structures, from smoothies to servings of mixed greens, permitted this individual to keep an assorted and supplement pressed diet while chasing after their wellness objectives.

An alternate point of view comes from somebody overseeing weight and zeroing in on generally prosperity. This singular offers their experience of integrating avocados into a decent eating regimen for weight the board. By embracing the satisfying properties of avocados, they found that it helped control their hunger and decrease unfortunate eating. The individual stresses the significance of part control and careful eating, featuring how avocados assumed an essential part in their weight reduction venture. Past the actual angles, they likewise examine the positive effect on their close to home prosperity, as the consideration of avocados gave pleasure and fulfillment to their dinners.

An exceptional individual story comes from a the parent advantages of avocados while acquainting strong food sources with their child. This singular offers the difficulties of tracking down supplement thick and agreeable choices for their youngster. Avocados arose as an answer, giving fundamental supplements to development and improvement. The parent considers the comfort of avocados as a convenient and effectively mashable nourishment for their child. The positive encounters with avocados during outset stretched out into youth, where the youngster fostered an inclination for healthy and supplement rich food varieties, setting an establishment for a solid relationship with sustenance.

For some's purposes, the avocado way of life is about something other than sustenance — it's an excursion of investigating culinary inventiveness. A self-declared food lover shares their experience of exploring different avenues regarding avocados in different recipes. From avocado-based dressings and dunks to integrating it into sweets, this singular features the adaptability of avocados in the kitchen. They express the way in which the avocado way of life turned into a wellspring of euphoria and motivation, igniting an energy for cooking and a recently discovered appreciation for new, entire food varieties. The individual additionally examines the social part of imparting avocado-roused dishes to loved ones, transforming feasts into essential and pleasant encounters.

An individual tribute comes from an individual overseeing explicit medical issue, like elevated cholesterol and irritation. This individual offers their excursion of embracing a heart-sound way of life, with avocados assuming a focal part in their dietary decisions. They examine the positive effect on their cholesterol levels, crediting it to the monounsaturated fats in avocados. Furthermore, the calming properties of avocados added to a decrease in joint agony and worked on generally portability. The individual underscores the significance of working intimately with medical services experts to fit dietary decisions to individual wellbeing needs.

An individual story likewise investigates the social meaning of avocados in unambiguous networks. This singular offers how avocados have been a conventional and treasured fixing in their family's culinary legacy. They examine the job of avocados in social festivals, as well as regular feasts, cultivating a feeling of association with their underlying foundations. The individual considers how the avocado way of life isn't simply an individual decision yet a social practice went down through ages, adding to a rich and significant food culture.

One strong tribute comes from a person who confronted difficulties connected with emotional wellness. This individual examines their excursion of defeating nervousness and melancholy and the job that dietary changes, including the joining of avocados, played in their recuperation. They share how avocados, with their supplement content and mind-set balancing out properties, turned into a major piece of their emotional well-being technique. The individual underscores the significance of comprehensive prosperity and how the avocado way of life, combined with other positive propensities, added to an extraordinary and elevating experience.

The encounters partook in these individual stories and tributes highlight the multi-layered effect of embracing the avocado way of life. From actual wellbeing and wellness to culinary imagination and mental prosperity, people articulate how avocados have turned into a positive power in their lives. These stories feature the flexibility of avocados to different inclinations and requirements, pursuing them an adaptable and open decision for a large number of people.

It's fundamental to perceive that these individual stories address individual encounters, and the advantages ascribed to the avocado way of life might change from one individual to another. While avocados offer various wholesome benefits, factors like generally speaking eating regimen, way of life, and individual medical issue assume a part in molding the results of integrating avocados into one's daily schedule.

These individual stories likewise highlight the more extensive idea of the avocado way of life as not only a dietary decision however an all encompassing way to deal with prosperity. Past the dietary angles, people address the close to home, social, and social components of their encounters with avocados. This all encompassing point of view lines up with the general topic of thinking about wellbeing and prosperity in a complete and interconnected way.

All in all, the individual stories and tributes of people who have embraced the avocado way of life give a rich embroidery of encounters that reach out a long ways past the nourishing domain. From wellness devotees and weight chiefs to guardians and those exploring explicit medical issue, these stories enlighten the different manners by which avocados have decidedly impacted lives. The avocado way of life arises as a dynamic and versatile methodology, offering medical advantages as well as happiness, innovativeness, and a feeling of association with culture and custom. As these individual stories illustrate, the avocado way of life is an excursion of revelation, change, and comprehensive prosperity.

www.ingramcontent.com/pod-product-compliance
Lightning Source LLC
LaVergne TN
LVHW010216070526
838199LV00062B/4621